ANTI-INFLAMMATORY DIET COOKBOOK:

Understanding Anti-Inflammatory Foods to Lead a Healthy Lifestyle

Mark Arizona

TABLE OF CONTENTS

Esqueixat Cod
Spinacas A La Catalana
Eggs To La Mallorquina
Eggs in Lemon
Break Cauliflower
Bread Soup
Beans
Puré De Calabacín
Xató
<u>Niçoise Salad</u>
Grilled Prawns
Quick Escaliveda
Steam Mussels
Potatoes With Peppers
Cold Tuna Cake
Garbanzos Al Wine
Soup / Fish Bracket
Samfaine
Mussels With Spicy Sauce
Pure Potatoes
Pasta Salad
Macaroni With Meat Sauce
Tempered Salad
Vegetables
Berenjena, Alcachofa, and Calabacín Fritos
Ground Beans With Potatoes
Russian Salad
White Wine Tellin
Tomato and Onion Salad
Roasted Potatoes
Vinegar Potatoes
Angulas or Surimi
Sealed Salad
Puree of Peas
Girgolas
Calçots

Turkey With Vegetables
Tigers (Breaded Mussels)
Tomato and Cucumber Salad With Yogurt Sauce
Mussels in Escabeche
Lobsters
Niscalo (Rovelló) A La Brasa
Jurel's Escabeche
Cheap Marisco Splash
Xavier Sauce
Artichoke
Cabañil Garlic
Alioli

Chapter 6 - Mains

Stripe With Green Sauce
Lamb With Beans
Lentils
Sepia With Potatoes
Rice With Fried Egg
Rice
Mixed Rice
Rice With Cod
Estofado Rabbit
Vegetable Rice
Chicken With Pinion
Loin With Tomato
Macaroni
Filled Chicken
Tenderloin
Filled Calamares
Cod With Aioli
Grilled Lamb
Poultry Fillets
Lamb to the Oven
Wrapped Honey

Sea Treat
Zarzuela Fish and Marisco Express
Baked Salmonetes
Coca
Rajada Delete
Duck
Snails With Ham
Russian Bistec
Rabbit With Vinagreta De Piñones
Ham Croquettes
Fideuà
Musaka

Chapter 7 - Desserts

Rice With Milk
Macedonia of Fruits
Strawberries in English Cream
Pan Greixonera
Floating Island
Pineapple Brush and Catalan Cream
Pears and Wine
Sweet Milk
Traditional Greixonera

Chapter 8 - Drinks

Bleeding
Chufa Horchata

Conclusion

INTRODUCTION

Congratulations on purchasing *Anti-inflammatory Diet Cookbook,* and thank you for doing so.

There are plenty of books on this subject on the market, thanks again for choosing this one! Every effort was made to ensure it is full of as much useful information as possible. Please enjoy!

Our ancestors were generally peasant people, the majority of the inhabitants of the planet in the last century, lived in small communities, the classic major or minor towns and the cities were reserved for the few. Now it is the opposite, most of us are grouped in great cities that sometimes become unbearable, but that ends up getting into our environment and way of life.

The meals of the towns have always been reputed to be very nutritious, however those of the cities were also reputed to be very light to know what our ancestors ate, we must go back to times before the transfer of the people to the cities, and they depended a lot on the environment where the population of these inhabitants was found. As we are dealing with the Anti-inflammatory diet, we are going to talk about the generalized customs of these peoples that live around the Mediterranean Sea, and what has been called the Anti-inflammatory diet. In fact, the Anti-inflammatory diet differs from the rest of other diets by not having excess calories and always taking advantage of the products of the land.

CHAPTER 1 – INTRODUCTION TO ANTI-INFLAMMATORY DIET

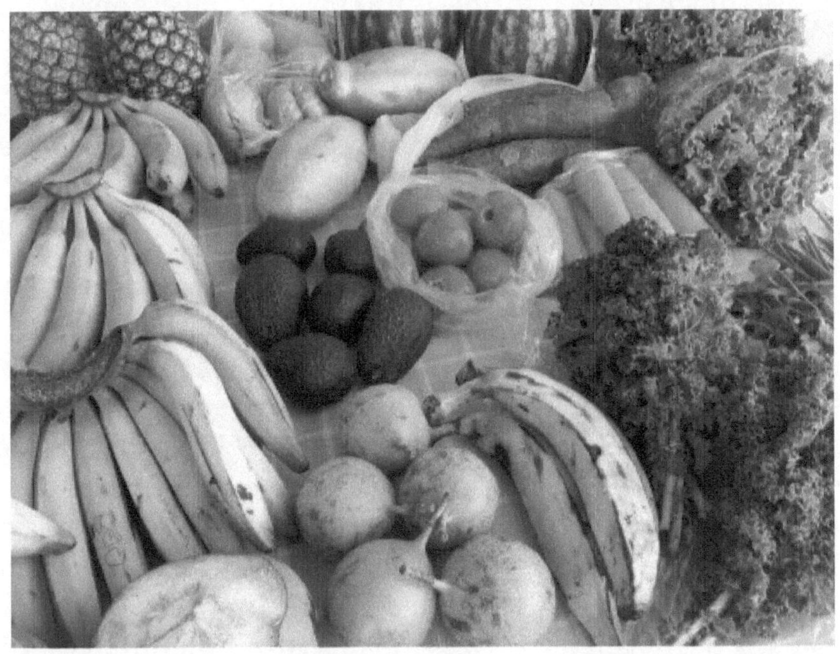

A classic Anti-inflammatory diet has always been based on what raised the land and the classic pig that each family killed in winter, so there are varieties in the Anti-inflammatory diets, and although small, they are worth considering. There is also a way to cook food in each part of the Anti-inflammatory, but it has something in common, and that is that the Anti-inflammatory diet uses many spices generally, abundant in salt and sometimes spicy, it is known that heat dehydrates and therefore Anti-inflammatory peoples use sometimes strong spices, as this allows them to drink much more water than not doing so. As an example, I will say that in India, where the weather is extremely hot and humid at the same time, the bodies need a lot of water to avoid dehydration, and that is the reason that their inhabitants expose when they are criticized for very spicy foods.

They say that if not, food would not allow them to drink water, and without it in the middle of the weather they have, they would become dehydrated. The same happens in the Anti-inflammatory where spices and spicy are used, although it must be said that spicy is not abused as it is done in India. The reason is that in the Anti-inflammatory, we have hot but not always humid climates, although it is necessary to recognize certain humid Anti-inflammatory regions and that at the same time are the ones that use the spicy spice.

People had varied customs according to the time in their meals, that is, in winter they ate many legumes and pork derivatives, as well as cereals, and in summer they ate many vegetables mainly in the form of salads and barely ate pork derivatives but increased consumption of the fruits of the time, these norms if they were practical all the Anti-inflammatory regions, and it was good norm that they ate like this. In the dietary norms, it is advised by the great specialists that the ideal is to eat foods of the time and of the land, something that our ancestors did; therefore, they managed to have their health much more balanced than we have today. Today you can and do eat any food at any time of the year, thanks to the greenhouses and the powerful refrigerators and freezers, this allows us to have any food at any time, but that does not mean that it is adequate or good for the human being. Therefore we have to let nature act and not do it for us. In the cases that we want to overcome nature, then we will pay the bill of not having understood our behavior, with a disease, since what has no logic will never have it; it is impossible for nature to do things halfway, she who is wise, makes every moment we have what is suitable for our organic balance.

We do not have to forget that if we follow in an orderly way what nature breeds in each era, we will realize that in the analysis of those foods, we will see the vitamins and minerals that we need at each moment, therefore, it has always been said that nature is wise, it is indeed comforting to know that there is someone without us or our family members who care about our wellbeing. Nature gives us our needs at all times, but of course, we must let it act on its own, we cannot make it unbalanced, because, with this, we will only be our victims, as an example I will say: The human being has a lot of need for vitamin C in spring more than in any other time of the year, and nature gives it to us through fruit, strawberry has 90% of vitamin C, and this fruit is logically Anti-inflammatory, it is normal that in Spring let's eat a lot of strawberries. In this and following the example, I will say, the human body has a lot of need for vitamin C in spring in summer, still having it but much less and gives us the melon with 30% and the peaches with 8%.

I am comparing only Anti-inflammatory fruits, since others may have more or less vitamin C, but they are not Anti-inflammatory, in autumn the organism is in need of this vitamin again, but that need is not as great as in spring and that is when it begins to be oranges that contain 55% of this vitamin, in winter the needs are equal to those of autumn, and that is why the orange is maintained throughout that time; therefore we have covered our vitamin C needs, if we follow the rules of nature and we eat what she gives us in each moment. This example of Vitamin C can also be translated to other vitamins, minerals, or proteins, in any of the ways, you just have to follow the mandates of nature.

CHAPTER 2 – ESSENTIAL FOODS

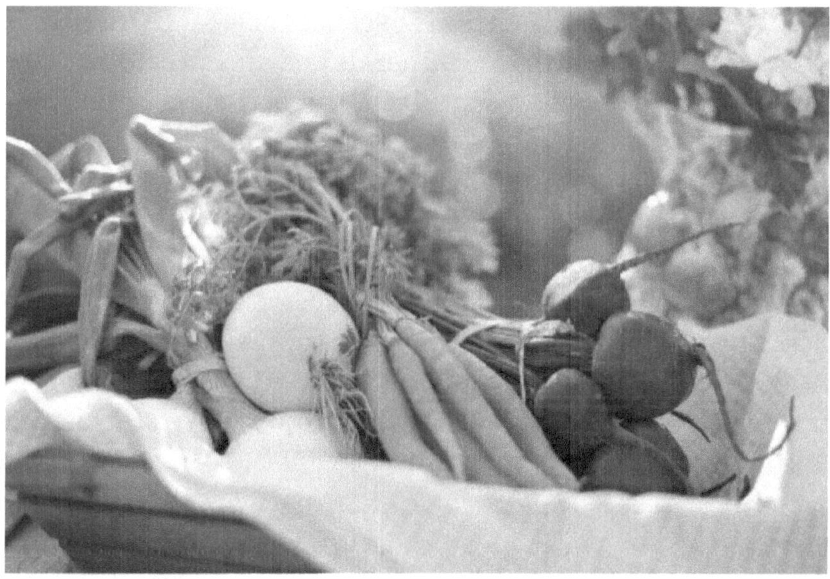

It has always been said that bread is an essential food for the Anti-inflammatory and it is true, this is given because it is the first food that human beings properly digest after breast milk has some essential amino acids such as tryptophan that In the absence of it, the human being falls into important endogenous depressions. Therefore it is a great food that nourishes and causes some proteins to be synthesized. What should be taken into account is to eat bread in an integral way, that is, as nature gives us, we cannot, in this case, rectify what she believes us; A refined bread does not contain the nutrients that humans need, and all they have is a large amount of starch, which will cause the body to be loaded with cholesterol and other cardiovascular problems. As we say bread is important, but also other cereals are for example rice, corn, rye, oats, barley, and others, we already know that Eastern people do not eat wheat cereal and if they eat it from rice, I will have to expose that rice is very similar to wheat and that is why the Orientals assimilated it instead of wheat as we Westerners did, but there are other towns such as Peru, Colombia, Venezuela, etc.

They do not eat wheat or rice cereal, and that is why they do not have deficiencies, and this is because they eat corn, corn has very rich properties in some minerals and amino acids, and this allows some proteins to be fixed and some of them transformed into other minerals that are not ingested directly as is the case with calcium. Do not forget that nature gives us what we need and also adapts it to our habitable environment; for this reason, it is necessary that we always take into account the food of the time and the terrain. This means that a person who lives in the Anti-inflammatory will be better off eating wheat cereal will do better with rice, and South Americans will do better with corn, etc. But when a Chinese comes to live in the Anti-inflammatory, it must be coupled to the customs of here and not theirs, just as if an Anti-inflammatory were to live in South America or the East, it must be coupled to the food customs that these people have, or otherwise, it may have important health deficiencies. I say again that nature knows why it should do things.

If we analyze carefully, we will realize that human beings have an anatomically prepared mouth to grind, our teeth are prepared mainly based on molars, and that is why the most important food after breast milk for us are cereals, our mouth has several molars, that is mill wheels to crush the grain, which really shows us the steps of our first food needs. It is important to observe how our ancestors did take this into account, then, they were not wrong in this food aspect, therefore, it is very clear that the first food that humans need after breast milk is cereals, they are great nutrients for us, and that is why they have been known since ancient times as food for human beings.

Our ancestors ate them in all their meals, but mainly at breakfast, now it is also about doing the same, what happens is that neither in the form nor in the content has anything to do what we do now with what they did before , and the truth is that it is known that what we do now is not correct, but if we have to eat as they did before it would not be right for us today, that is, those ancestors of ours ate a great dish in the morning of crumbs, (as we know wheat cereal in the form of bread or flour, cooked with olive oil and sometimes some crooked "pork bacon"), is excess calories that this food has, is clearly poorly digested by us , since now we do not do what those of our ancestors, who were going to work in the field hard, now we are generally going to work in a factory or office and almost always those jobs are not great efforts, therefore, you could not burn the calories that a bowl of crumbs has.

Therefore, it is necessary to observe what we do now, usually a coffee with milk and some cookies (refined cereal), seeing thus, we see the great difference that exists between the plate of crumbs and coffee with milk and cookies. The first was correct for our ancestors since their work made them spend a lot of energy, the second is the current thing that although the work does not make us spend as many energies it does not have logic as we do, for several reasons: the first reason is that Coffee is a stimulant that tremendously affects the nervous and cardiovascular system, the second is milk, food for calves and not for humans, none of the components of animal milk, are adapted so that human beings can digest it Therefore, we cannot say that animal milk is good for human beings; but it also has another great defect, that milk when mixed with coffee, produces a digestive acidity that causes the food to become anti-food, and then to top it off, we eat wheat biscuits but refined, that is, they have all taken away the nutrients when refining the flour, at least our ancestors ate unrefined flour, that is to say integral with all their nutrients; as we see what our ancestors did was good for their time, what we do now it is not good either for our time or to nourish ourselves, therefore, we have to make a true Anti-inflammatory diet adapted to our time but that nourishes us, so many poorly nourished children with cholesterol excesses have never been seen in medical consultation very high, when children are mainly the number one eating cereals, what happens is that now these cereals are refined, and it is not possible that it nourishes them and on the contrary if it raises their cholesterol rates, lowers their defenses and makes them be drifting from health, when they don't have one thing, they have another, this hardly happened before.

If we add to these other ways of life, heavily polluted cities, food prepared, and preserved with preservative products that are sometimes carcinogenic; we have all the ballots for us to be chronically ill for life.

And I wonder, shouldn't it be that there are many sick people to do important business with health? The customs that we have been adapting are sick, and therefore we have to make a peaceful and psychological revolution within us considering whether it really suits us to follow the path we are going.

Commenting on the breakfasts they made and what we do, we have to come to the conclusion that the former could not do us good now because of our way of working, the latter does not do us good because they are not nutrients, then it is necessary to make nutrient breakfasts and they would be very easy to do: in these current times we have to demand that houses that are dedicated to food preparations, especially "quality", not refining food and much less cereals, cereals are an important source of Nutrients provided they are ingested integrally; otherwise we are eating something false, something that we think nourishes us, but it is not true, and in the long run we will be sick from poor nutrition. Do not confuse filling the stomach with nutrition, one thing is different from the other, the stomach is filled even if it is garbage, but good nutrition can only be made by a food that is complete, for all this, we have to understand that cereals Wholegrains are good for making our breakfasts a cup of whole grains mixed with water and sweetened with honey, and a digestive tea would be a good breakfast, there are varieties that later when we recommend the appropriate diets for the modern human being we will expose, but it is simple Formula is adequate and will be well nourished.

Many will tell us that milk is missing and I say again that animal milk is not the food of the human being, it is the food of calves, I know that they will say that if you do not drink milk we will lack calcium, because it is not true, since it is shown that people who drink a lot of milk are first candidates for osteoporosis, osteoarthritis and all degenerative bone diseases, therefore it is not true; The reason why that person who drinks so much milk and lacks calcium, is because calcium is not fixed in the body directly, can only be fixed by the action of other minerals such as magnesium, manganese or silicon, so In people who should be treated for a lack of calcium, it is of no use that we fill them with calcium, since they will never fix it, however, if we give them adequate doses of magnesium, manganese or silicon, they will form an extraordinary calcium of Great quality and will recover the wear. This happens, because the organism only fixes nutrients by means of transmutation, that is, when transmuting it chooses among those nutrients, those that are suitable for its balance.

It is also shown that the body fixes much more nutrients if they are eaten in small quantities, but many more times a day, which means that not by getting fed up we will have better nutrients or in more quantity, on the contrary, nutrients they are fixed in the body when they have accumulated in small doses, large quantities are lost and expelled in the feces, therefore, it would be advisable to eat between 5 to 7 times a day in small quantities, that is, that the all the calories of the day are distributed among those meals that we are going to make. In this way food is not only better used, but also the insulin curve produced by food is much more balanced when small meals are made and, in more times, which makes it clear that diabetic patients should eat in this way and not only in two or three meals a day.

In the West, there is a very entrenched custom that is to eat a lot of bread at all meals, and after mealtimes, whole wheat bread is a good nutrient, but like all flours it contains excess carbohydrates, and It makes you fat, let alone refined white bread, which has become almost entirely starchy, fattens much more and does not nourish, so it is necessary to know that whole wheat bread even if it is a good nutrient we cannot abuse it if not we want to be obese, now our jobs do not make us burn energy barely and the excesses cause us obesity, therefore, be careful with bread, Italian pasta, etc. Flour derivatives and much more if the flour has been refined, one or two slices of whole wheat bread, and if it is possible that it is toasted, it will be adequate so that we do not fall into obesity.

All food the first thing you have to do in digestion, is to nourish, the food that does not nourish, fills the stomach, but it is useless, and in the long run, we will have great food deficiencies thinking that we have eaten well and even that we have eaten too much.

We have to look at some villages, some malnourished for lack of food (hunger) and others for excess refined food; In the first aspect, the African peoples take the palm when it comes to poor nutrition due to lack of generalized food, and in the second aspect it is the North Americans who take the palm, the excess of food and, above all, food refined, it makes them beat the whole world in being poorly fed, there is usually in the USA. Many are obese due to the excesses of malnourished foods and loaded with carbohydrates: it seems incredible that a country like this that cares a lot about research, is not worried about this aspect that is very common among them. Returning to the aspect of the food that our ancestors ate, we have already seen how they ate breakfast, and now we are going to see how they had lunch, we generally know that they were peasant beings and that they worked in the field.

For the same reason, the midday meal could not be done between 1 p.m. and 3 p.m. and hot, they took to the field raw food that was the general base at that time, that is, around 1 p.m. they used to eat and what they did was make a very varied salad of several vegetables example: lettuce, tomato, carrot, radishes, etc., and almost always mixed or dried tuna or cod, with that they were completing the proteins, and others what they did was eat the Salad with the vegetables alone and after eating a piece of ham, bacon, sausage, cod, or some other sausage. If we compare this with what we eat today, it has nothing to do with it. Today a very strong meal is made at noon and usually somewhat late between 2 pm and 3 pm, and this meal in most cases is composed of two or three dishes, some of them being hot and another fried. This custom does not now have all the peoples of the world, but mainly the Anti-inflammatory, since if we consider the Saxons, we will see how they continue to make a very smooth lunch at 1:00 p.m. and dinner is usually done at 6:00 p.m. 19 hours, but the Anti-inflammatory people who are those who occupy us in this treaty, we are like this, we eat too much and somewhat late, these customs should have remained like that of our ancestors, although and since it can be done by work, do strong food at noon, let's do something earlier and less loaded, and especially something that we should not forget, is to do what our ancestors did, eat a vegetable salad as a first course, the second could be the hot avocado and there should never be a third party, never drink dessert coffee, it is shown that coffee delays digestion, take chamomile tea, pulley, green anise, etc., since these are digestive and will help us to digest better.

At lunch you should eat whole wheat bread, one or two toasted slices, it is also shown that toasted bread is much more digestive than simply cooked, so whenever we can we should eat whole wheat and toasted bread, but we will never abuse it , we already know that it contains many carbohydrates and they excessively make you fat. We must clarify that carbohydrates are very necessary for humans, they, together with fats, form organic energy to have enough strength for life, but the excesses of some and others will make us fat. I insist that now we do not burn the excess calories as our ancestors did working hard in the field, now most of us are working sitting eight hours and although the mind wears a lot of caloric energy accumulate and make us fat.

CHAPTER 3 – MAINTAINING A HEALTHY HABIT

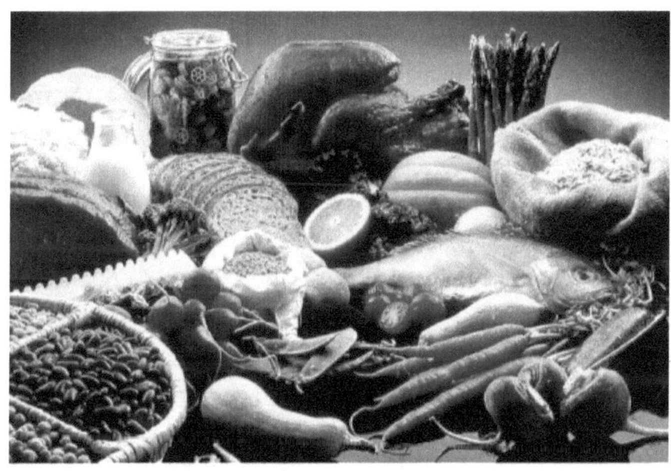

Our elders had a very good habit, they ate fruit only between hours, that is to say in what we call mid-morning and mid-afternoon, that is to eat fruit intelligently, since the fruit of eating it as a dessert makes you gain weight, that's why you have to eat it outside of hours of meals, in separate digestions, but yes, eat it because it is very necessary, the vitamins they contain are very important for the fixation of proteins and other nutrients and especially for organic cleaning, fruits are very cleansing and make The body eliminates its toxins properly some of these vitamins participate in the formation of red blood cells and in the formation of iron as is the case with vitamin C, but all of them have very important specific functions in the body.

The fruit is good to the point that we must make a day of a fruit meal once a week, that is, at each meal of the day a different type of fruit so as not to mix them together, the fruits when mixed, produce acidity in the blood, only the apple is the fruit that could be mixed with the others without this happening for that reason, the fruits should not be mixed with each other, there is also a lot of variety and at each meal we can use a different type of fruit, if well it is necessary that in each epoch they eat their own. We know that now we can find any fruit at any time of the year, by the art of greenhouses, but that is not normal, if this were normal, nature would have given us all kinds of fruits at any time of the year. Each season has its fruit, and the organism needs it according to nature, it will also be good to put into practice fruit fasting, especially in spring and autumn, which are the two strongest seasons of the year and when the body needs to purify much more and prepare for what comes up.

Fasting must always be controlled, it can be done three days, one week and nine days, and these days we will eat only fruit of the time, that is to say, no other, it is about doing a strong cleaning and also charging the batteries. Therefore, it should be made of a type of fruit only and adequate at the time; In Spring, fasting can be done with strawberries and in Autumn it must be done with grapes, others can also be used, but they must be fruits of the time, that is, nature gives them to us at that time of year. If we do a fast, days before we must prepare, that is, do not cut off with normal food and suddenly we get into fasting, that creates some anxiety in some people and they cannot finish the fasting they had proposed, it is better to enter two or three days before, lowering the type of food we eat, that are softer and that vegetables and fruits are present in them, and so when we enter the days of fasting based on fruits we will tolerate it well and not we will have anxiety, the exit of the fast should be done the same as the entrance, not start another day of fasting to eat everything, since we could have wasted time with fasting, do the same as to enter two or three days to eat mainly vegetables and fruits and some cereal, but the proteins above all of the meat and fish should not be eaten in those days, the fact of being several days without eating any kind of food, nothing happens, although in this case, it is for doing one organic cleaning, that is what we will achieve, cleaning our body, so that we can enter the season with strength and vital energies.

Our ancestors took into account these two seasons that we have been commenting on, spring and autumn, and generally, what they did at the beginning of these two seasons was to purge themselves with rectal oil or with carabane water. Both purgatives very effective, and that would be suitable also to do them today if we do not do the fasting of fruits indicated above. A purge twice a year is practically essential for our body to function well, it is the same as if comparatively the clothes we put on do not wash it, there would come a time when it would be dirty and damaged, so we take care of it, wash it, iron, and we sew if it has some ripping and all this to keep it in shape, however, little we care about our own organism, it seems as if we do not care whether it is damaged or not.

In this also our elders saw more clearly these aspects with respect to organic cleaning, therefore, my recommendation cannot be other than either we do a fruit fast twice a year, or purge twice a year, purge more effective is the liver cleanse, that is to say the toxic filter, if we clean this filter we will be able to live with less organic problems, comparatively like the filter of a car, if the car is dirty, the car malfunctions and if the car is clean car runs well, the same goes for the body, the filter is that the liver must always be clean and for this at the entrance of the strong seasons such as Spring and Autumn, we should do an organic cleaning with a liver purge mainly, this purge should be done as follows: at bedtime the night Have her drink half a glass of olive oil, half a glass of lemon juice and together a glass of water-boiling tea with a tablespoon of senna leaves, everything is taken together, and that night you don't have dinner. With this purge, we have all the security that we have cleaned the liver and that the filter is again to do its job properly.

As we can also see in this, our ancestors were taller than us, we have neglected many aspects because they have led us to believe that they were not good, and I ask myself again, would it not be that we were not interested in our body being healthy?

Taking up the food of our elders, we will see how the dinners they made were very different from us, they used to dine at sunset more or less, that is to say at dusk in winter and in Summer, that is when they returned from work in the field, and in those hours they ate the hot plate, considering eating many legumes. The legume is a regulatory food, this is because in its composition it has an adequate proportions of the three immediate principles of food, that is, they contain proteins, fats, and carbohydrates and also contain them in the balance we need, that is, 15% of proteins, 25% of fats and 65% of carbohydrates, which are the appropriate proportions in which we must eat to eat foods that are nutrients, otherwise we will be eating foods that do not nourish us. As we see the dinners they made are in hours and content similar to those still made by the Anglo-Saxons, we lost those customs when moving from the countryside to the cities and now we usually eat dinner from 9pm to 11pm, also strong and we go to bed at most 24 hours, with which we go to bed doing the digestion, and the moment we fall asleep the digestion slows down so that it is almost impossible to do it. That is why it has been written and said that there are many tombs full of good dinners, and this saying really has, if we take into account our form and hours of dinner, for this reason, we are in a very big mistake in several ways in the way and In the content, mealtimes cannot be crazy so that digestion can be done, if a digestion is not done, we will not be nourished or healthy.

It is convenient to observe how our Europeans brothers do this, that although analyzed is how our ancestors did it, that is why there is no choice but to change the meal times to the customs of yesteryear since it is shown that they are the logical hours of eating and not as we Spaniards do. Breakfast should be made from 8 to 9 hours, lunch should be made from 13 to 14 hours and dinner from 20 to 21 hours and never later, since otherwise the digestion of food will not be done well, if We are hungry between those hours, the logical thing is that we take advantage and eat fruit, the fruit has very interesting nutrients for our body and they are very necessary. It is convenient that we go back in these customs, it is not possible to maintain illogical schedules, our bodies need nutrients to be able to continue living with health, but we strive to do everything against the current, and we understand that the body has to endure what they throw, because dear reader, the body endures while it can, and then gets sick, because what is not understood in our con-science we will suffer in our physical body, suffering, and suffer-ing.

It would be much better if we learned to prevent and thus not have to cure, it would be to make true preventive medicine, or perhaps dear reader thinks that preventive medicine is to take medications to not get sick, well, no, for many medications that one takes, when the organism He doesn't need them, they won't help; the body will get sick in every way, and it will have been useless to cram ourselves with pills, capsules, drops, etc. The body will get sick because, in reality, what will really serve as a preventive is an adequate meal that nourishes it.

It is time to eat again in the hours of our ancestors; we also do not stop saying that we are Europeans, but our brothers Euro-peans have a few hours and customs of feeding very different from us, let's make at least one of our diet Anti-inflammatory.

CHAPTER 4 - THE IMPORTANCE OF MEDITERRANEAN **Food**

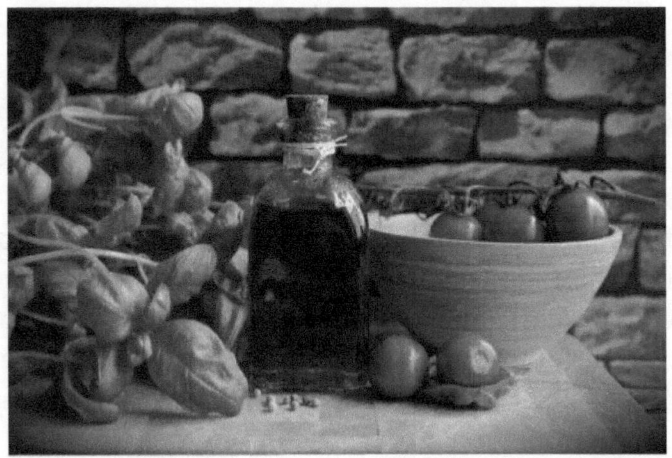

The first thing we should know in this regard is how the three immediate principles act, and for them, we see their different forms of food breakdown:

FOOD AND NUTRITIONAL SUBSTANCES

Through food, we naturally present nutritional substances such as legumes, fish, meat, fruits, eggs, etc. Each food consists of six nutritional substances in different proportions of each other; being these six substances:

- Protein
- Fats
- Carbohydrates (starches and sugars, among others).
- Vitamins
- Minerals
- Water

WHAT ARE CALLED IMMEDIATE PRINCIPLES?

In the domestic environment, meals are calculated with foods of various types: meat, eggs, fish, vegetables, cereals, legumes, etc., to introduce adequate diets, the dietitian, has in mind the immediate composition of those foods.

FOOD COMPOSITION AND FUNCTIONAL CLASSIFICATION THEREOF

In each food, one of those elements predominates, this being what makes each food have value to fulfill a certain function:

- In meats, proteins predominate
- In fish, proteins predominate
- In eggs, proteins predominate
- In milk, proteins and calcium predominate
- In cheese, proteins and calcium predominate
- In vegetables, vitamins predominate
- In fruits, vitamins predominate
- In bread, flour, rice, carbohydrates predominate
- In oil, butter, bacon, fats predominate
- In legumes, there is a certain balance of everything.

ROLE OF EACH IMMEDIATE PRINCIPLE

Proteins:

They form the muscles, "the framework" of the bones, and in general, all the cells of the organism.
That is, protein-rich foods have a tissue-forming function in the body and are therefore essential in the growing season and also necessary in the adult to repair tissues.

The best quality proteins are found in those of vegetable origin, in soybeans, and in those of animal origin in eggs; Those of animal origin, being important, must take into account their toxic content.

Fats:

They provide energy to the body and form adipose tissue; that is, they provide calories and accumulate them, which, when transformed into energy, produces strength to work.

Carbohydrates:

Carbohydrates are found mainly in; sweets, flours, pasta, bread, corn, etc. They also provide an amplitude of calories and energy. Foods par excellence of calories, fats, and carbohydrates, are called energy foods.

Minerals:

Some are part of the bones, as is the case with calcium, others with blood hemoglobin, as is the case with iron, and so each of them has its organic function.

Minerals should not be taken without a prescription, since, if so, you can fall into mineral malnutrition without wanting to; there are minerals that to be fixed must be accompanied by others and in fair proportions; such is the case of calcium, that to fix it well, it is necessary to take it with magnesium, and in proportions of 2 parts of calcium per 1 of magnesium, otherwise it is not fixed well; others are essential in allergies, such as zinc; others are key in cardiovascular diseases, as is the case with selenium, and so, each of them, has its effects on the body.

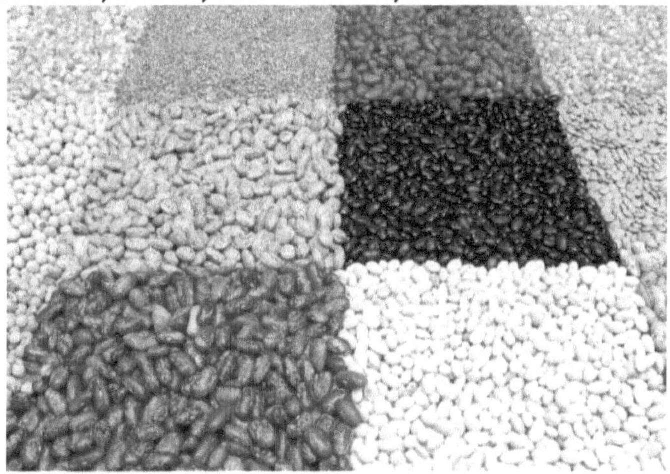

Vitamins:

Vitamins are part of the ferments that regulate the use of other substances; Like minerals, vitamins have very important effects for the body; Such is the case of some of them such as B, which is purifying in all its concepts, we all know that from the vitamin B range there are from B1 to B15 and some of them have specific functions such as the case of B1 that is vital in allergies and B6 with extraordinary effects on eyesight and lumbociatics, also B12 has important effects on eyesight and lumbociática such is the case of vitamin E, essential for cardiovascular disease, the A to maintain the night vision, the D3 for the good calcium swab, especially in the bone mass, etc.

Foods rich in minerals and vitamins have a quality function in the diet.

It does not provide "quantity" or calories, but they are essential to maintain a perfect state of health. Both vitamins and minerals, have a regulatory function, acting as controllers to use the remaining nutrients, so, by the action of them, proteins will form the muscle, fats, and carbohydrates are burned to provide the precise calories that will move the organic engine.

From all of the above, we deduce that the nutrients can be:

1. plastics (proteins and some minerals)

- Milk
- Cheese
- Meat
- Fish
- Eggs
- Legumes (partially, due to their protein content)

2. energy (fats and carbohydrates)

- cereals (bread, flour, rice, etc.)
- fats (oils, bacon, butter, etc.)
- legumes (partially because of their carbohydrate content)

3. regulators (vitamins and some minerals)

- fruits
- vegetables
- legumes (due to their content partially in vitamins and minerals)

We can ask ourselves, what are each immediate principles?

Carbohydrates:

They are substances composed of carbon, oxygen, and hydrogen; we are the latter two in the same proportion as in water, that is, H2O, so they are called hydrates.

Plants synthesize them from carbon dioxide and water. Man and animals receive them by eating them in plant foods.

But they can synthesize them from fat proteins. In the digestion of vegetables in the digestive system, carbohydrates are attacked by various ferments and eventually degrade to glucose. Glucose circulates in the blood, and thanks to a hormone called insulin, it penetrates the cells, where it burns (oxidized), producing energy.

It's important to know:

- For every gram of carbohydrates that is burned, 4 calories are produced.
- Most glucose is transformed into fat; therefore, bread, sugar, rice, etc. They gain weight.

Foods rich in carbohydrates are:

- Bread, flour, Italian pasta, rice, etc.
- Sugar, candy, buns, cookies.
- Legumes (beans, lentils, chickpeas, beans) but not so soy.

From this knowledge, we deduce that in the diabetic patient (in which insulin is lacking), these foods should be reduced because glucose by not penetrating the cells and not being used, it accumulates in the blood and is eliminated in the urine.

However, it must be taken into account; some of these foods are necessary for diabetics:

Legumes (lentils) because of its high iron content, for better blood hemoglobin; Soy, which has a low carbohydrate content.

Fruits taking into account that sugar fructose is even recommended in these patients, provided they do not go up to 60 grams per day, which means that the diabetic should take into account not eating fruits that contain a higher percentage of glucose such as the following:

- Bananas
- Grapes
- Apricots, cherry, and cherry
- Avocado
- Pineapple
- Figs
- Chestnuts
- Kiwis and all the tropical fruits

Fats:

Like carbohydrates, they are made up of carbon, oxygen, and hydrogen, and their main function is to provide caloric energies.

They can carry some vitamins (fat-soluble) and certain essential fatty acids in the diet. Solid (food) or liquid fats (oils) are attacked in the digestive system by ferments and converted into simpler substances that are then absorbed and transported by the blood to the cells.

When burned, each gram of fat provides 9 calories.

Fatty foods are:
- Some cheeses, bacon, sausages, pork, turkey.
- Bluefish (although their fats are a great solvent of cholesterol
- Butter, margarine, oils.

The diet too high in fat produces obesity and cholesterol.

CHAPTER 5 - STARTERS AND APPETIZERS

POTATO TORTILLA

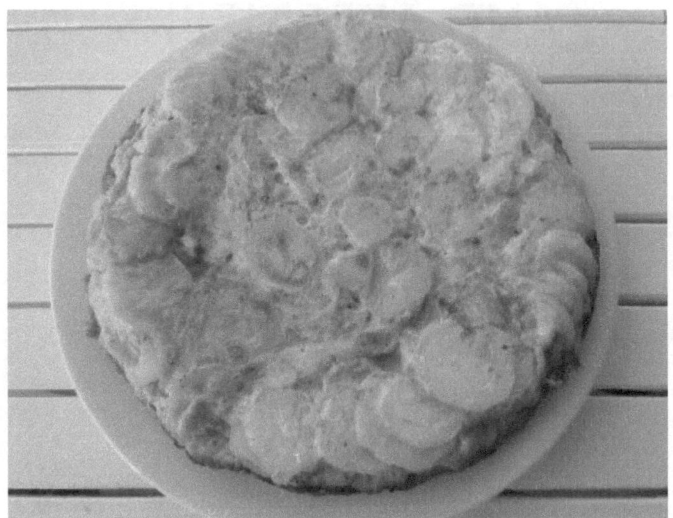

Ingredients for four / five people:
5-6 large potatoes
5 fresh eggs
olive oil
salt
large pan

Fill an anti-stick pan with plenty of oil up to about 1 finger.
Cut the potatoes into small squares or thin slices. It is important not to make the pieces too large to avoid long frying times. We throw the potatoes cut in the hot oil with salt. We place a lid to accelerate cooking, ensuring that the oil does not overheat (reduce the fire if appropriate). From time to time, we stir with a wooden spoon to homogenize the frying. When removing, we will try to make the lid open as little as possible to prevent water vapor from escaping. From time to time, we will try to press a piece of potato to see if it is soft enough. In general, the

frying is ready when the potatoes acquire a translucent hue, and some are lightly toasted (not burned).

We will beat 5 eggs by adding a little salt, and we will throw them on the potatoes so that the tortilla sets. If there is too much oil, it is better to take out the potatoes and put them in a separate container to remove the excess oil and then add the egg in "cold," stirring well so that the potatoes are completely soaked.

We add all the content to the pan allowing it to set while continuing to move it circularly to avoid burning or sticking the face of the tortilla we do not see. Before the entire visible part of the egg sets, we will place a ceramic plate that is approximately the size of the pan, press, and with a quick turn of the wrist, we will turn around. If all is well, the tortilla will remain on the plate. We will leave the pan on the fire again to slide the side of the tortilla that must be finished, and in a couple of minutes, the tortilla will be made.

Estimated time: 20 minutes

CHICKEN SOIL

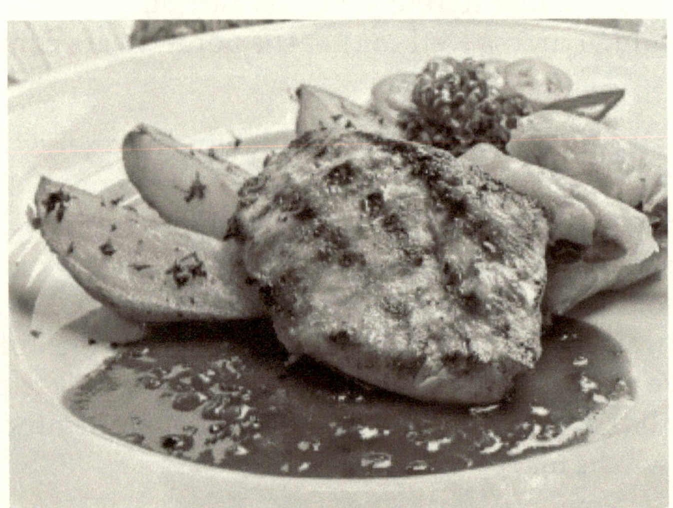

Chicken broth has a double utility: as a separate dish and as a base for other recipes instead of simply adding water. Even as an independent dish, it can be said that there are actually two: a slightly fatty soup and the product of the stew - potato, chick-pea, chicken, etc. The preparation of a chicken broth takes more than 30 minutes, but the longer duration is compensated with less work in the realization: you put all the ingredients in the pan and boil.

The ingredients may vary as they are not critical, although the usual ones are:

Potato (3 or 4)

Onion or Leek or a combination of both Celery and Chickpeas (250-400 grams), which can be cooked or better dried soaked from the previous day.

Chicken (a quarter, a breast, etc.)

Carrot (1 large)

Salt (two tablespoons)

Water
It is also possible to put a bay leaf or other aromatic herbs, although it is not essential.

We put in a large casserole (capable of containing 3 or 4 liters of water) all the ingredients. It is convenient to use large uncut potatoes, just like carrots. If the chickpeas are dry, we will put them at the beginning, but if they are cooked, we will add them almost at the end of cooking - otherwise, we run the risk of being undone.

Cover with water, if possible, bottled or filtered to remove impurities. We can use tap water, but then we must be careful, especially if we want a transparent broth to remove the impurities from the surface of the water with a spoon from time to time (this also happens with bottled or filtered water but in a lesser extent).

The cooking time is about 1 hour and a half. If everything went well, the potatoes will be broken or quite depleted as well as the chicken. That is good to some extent since the "philosophy" of the broth is that the nutrients of the elements that we have introduced pass into the water, but it is bad if we have spent in cooking and "killed" the nutrients we wanted. In any case, at the end of the cooking period, we will have a more or less thick broth and a solid residue consisting of chickpeas, potatoes, chicken, celery, etc. We will proceed to strain the broth to separate the liquid from the solid residue. Said residue can be consumed directly once cleaned of bones, although it is possible to indicate that naturally, because of the whole cooking process, it has lost much of its properties.

The broth is the basis for many possible applications. For example, you can make a soup by adding a tablespoon of rice or use some pasta for the same purpose. Particularly I like to keep the broth with part of the chicken meat that I place on each plate, accompanied by a little potato and chickpeas as a "stumble." That gives the feeling of homemade broth and not one of those broths obtained from concentrates.

If enough broth has been made, it is possible to replace the water of any dish (rice, pasta, vegetables) and give it a strong consistency. Unlike other broths, chicken does not mask the flavors, especially if we include onion instead of leek.

SIMPLE GARLIC SPAGHETTI

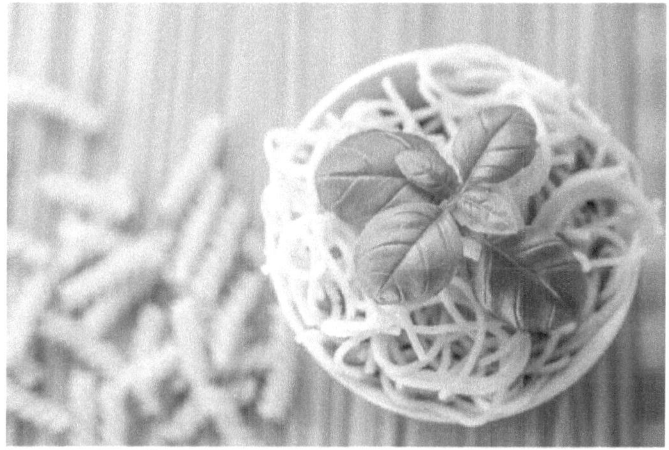

This dish requires less than 10 minutes of preparation.
We need:
Parsley dried or fresh spaghetti
Garlic
Grated cheese
virgin olive oil
If we start from dry spaghetti, we will take an adequate amount according to the number of diners. We must think that the weight of the pasta once cooked doubles approximately the original so that 250 grams will generate 500 grams of pasta. We will boil the spaghetti in boiling water something salty according to the manufacturer's instructions, to obtain pasta al dente or soft, according to our taste. Meanwhile, in a non-stick skillet with two tablespoons of olive oil, we will have browned a garlic head and added some dried or fresh parsley, chopped well. Once the pasta is cooked - between 7 and 10 minutes - we will quickly

transfer it to the pan and with a wooden spoon we will stir the garlic and parsley with the pasta, adding some more salt, so that after a minute of work we will observe that the pasta has absorbed the oil and all the parsley is dispersed by the pasta. Remove from heat and consume immediately, optionally with grated cheese.

FRENCH TORTILLA WITH CHEESE

This dish requires slightly less than five minutes of preparation.
Ingredients:
1 or 2 fresh eggs (as needed) Creamy grated cheese
Salt
virgin olive oil
In a small pan (20 cm in diameter, for example) non-stick, we put a tablespoon of virgin olive oil and heat.
Beat the eggs by adding a pinch of salt (remember that the cheese is already a salty product). We pour the mixture over the hot oil so that it expands on the surface of the pan like a crepe. In the center of the circle that will be formed, and before it sets, we will deposit the grated cheese. Then we will fold the "wings" of the tortilla over the grated cheese so that it takes a tubular shape. We will turn the tortilla to close the fold and finish curdling inside. If the dish has been well-cooked, the tortilla will have a slight cheese flavor that will accompany the egg.

WHITE FRENCH TORTILLA

A white tortilla is the one we make without the egg yolk. The reason for this procedure is to limit cholesterol intake, especially in those prone to hypertension or who already live the problem.

This dish requires slightly less than five minutes of preparation.

Ingredients:

1 or 2 fresh eggs (as needed)

Creamy grated cheese

Salt

virgin olive oil

In a small non-stick pan (20 cm in diameter, for example), we put a tablespoon of virgin olive oil and heat. We break the eggs and carefully collect the yolk in one of the sections while we are transferring the egg white to the other half and then pouring it into the plate.

Beat the egg whites by adding a pinch of salt or directly without salt, as the diner needs. We pour the mixture over the hot oil so that it expands on the surface of the pan like a crepe. Next, we will bend the "wings" of the tortilla on itself so that it takes a tubular shape. We will turn the tortilla to close the fold and finish curdling inside. Undoubtedly the tortilla will look whitish instead of the typical yellowish appearance.

MURCIAN SHARP

Murcian cuisine is a great unknown, encased between the gigantism of the Valencian and the Andalusian. This ignorance is a great injustice considering that the Murcian garden feeds all of Spain with the best vegetables, of which the Zarangollo is a good example in the use of them. If the name of this dish sounds like Chinese, it is a clear demonstration that the advertising department of Murcian gastronomy does not work too well. It is a dish that can be ready in a few minutes.

Ingredients:
3 or 4 large-medium zucchinis
4 large onion
6 eggs
virgin olive oil
salt

Zucchini are peeled and sliced. Fry in the oil together with the onion cut in julienne. Add salt and cover the casserole (this will generate water and not burn). When they are fried, they will be removed by placing them in a drainer to remove excess oil. It will be mixed with the eggs and put back in a pan until set. It is served as a first course. To give an idea, use a zucchini-onion pair per diner.

CREPES

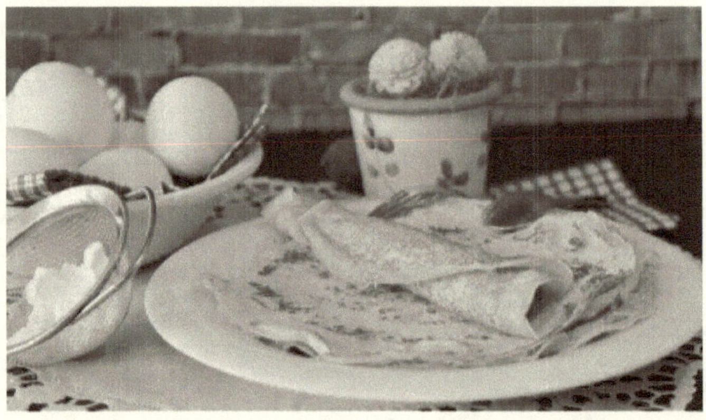

Crepes are a good support for both savory starters and desserts and are therefore very popular for breakfast: we can make a crepe roll filled with feta cheese and finish with a sweet crepe filled with fig jam. Although a distinction is usually made in all recipes between sweet and savory crepes, it is usually enough to make a single "salty" type leaving the salt point low so that the taste is neutral. Neutral crepes go well with salty and sweet ingredients, while sweets do not marry anything well with salty contents.

Ingredients:
3 glasses of wheat flour
1 glass of milk
2 eggs
3 tablespoons butter
1 pinch salt

Mix all the ingredients and beat them with the rod or electric mixer. The dough should be without lumps and neither very liquid nor solid (something like melted chocolate). If it is very dry, we will add milk, and if too liquid, we will rectify it with a little flour.

We place a nonstick skillet on the fire and heat it. With a little butter smear the bottom. Then, we take part of the dough with a saucepan of the employees to serve soup and place it in the center, stirring with a spatula to cover the entire bottom of the pan. When the edges begin to darken, we turn around (it would not hurt to add another bit of liquid butter) and let it be done. It is possible that the first crepe is only for testing since we may have to rectify the elasticity of the dough or the temperature of the plate.

Salty suggestions:
- Fill with feta cheese and ham
- Peppers, tuna and boiled egg
- Wild asparagus with cheese sauce

Sweet suggestions:
- Fill with fig jam
- Dulce de leche
- Chocolate and cream

POTAGE

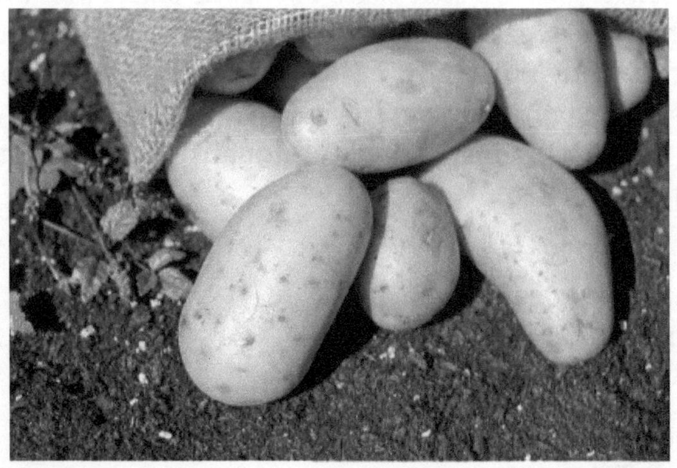

Again, this dish requires a preparation time greater than 30 minutes, but it has the great advantage that if we make a certain amount, we can consume it for several days and even freeze it, saving time "a posteriori." It is, therefore, an ideal dish to cook during the weekend and consume it throughout it.

Ingredients for 4 People (or 4 Portions):

Chickpeas (cooked or dried soaked the night before).
Potato (1 ½ potato per diner, medium type)
2 ripe tomatoes
1 onion
1 Green pepper
Chard or Spinach (200-400 grams)
Pumpkin (one piece) *
Dried beans soaked the night before (or cooked)
Salt
Olive oil
Water

*the pumpkin totally modifies the taste of the stew, and due to its sweetness, many people do not like it in the stew. Therefore, their employment is left to the discretion of each.

Unlike a simple broth, the stew incorporates a sauce that completely defines its aroma and flavor.

For the sofrito, we cut the onion and green pepper into very small pieces. We take a relatively large casserole (for 4 or 5 liters) and put oil in the bottom until covered with a very thin sheet. Heat and pour the green pepper to start frying. Then we toss the onion.

While we will take two tomatoes, we will peel them, we will open in half, and with the help of a teaspoon of coffee, we will remove the seeds. We will cut the tomatoes into very small pieces, and when the onion begins to brown, we will throw them to prevent burning (adding salt at this time will cause the vegetables to release even more water avoiding burning). A good stir-fry will be one in which the components are mixed until they acquire a uniform texture where the red color predominates, the aroma comes from the green pepper, and the base of the flavor is due to the onion.

Once the sofrito has the proper appearance and flavor, we will proceed to add the chickpeas, the dried beans (if the legumes were not dry but cooked, they would be added almost at the end of cooking). If we want to speed up the preparation, we will have heated 2 liters of water apart until almost boiling. With all the elements inside the casserole, with the exception of the vegetable and the potato, we will pour the water and stir with a wooden spoon or metallic ladle so that the sofrito is incorporated into the water. Cover the casserole.

As the mixture boils, we will check the hardness of the legumes. When they start to soften, we will add the potatoes cut into pieces.

We will continue over medium heat until we verify that we can stick a fork in the potatoes. It is time to add spinach. We will cover and let boil another half hour. If we want the broth to be thicker, we can take a piece of potato from the pan, crush it and return it to the liquid.

This dish is served with all the whole pieces in a deep dish with enough liquid to justify the use of the spoon. In some cases, some diners prefer to dress it with vinegar.

Another way to serve it is puree, but only if spinach has been used and does not chard. By passing all the ingredients through the blender, you get a thick dark green mash, which is really very tasty.

ISABEL FILLED EGGS

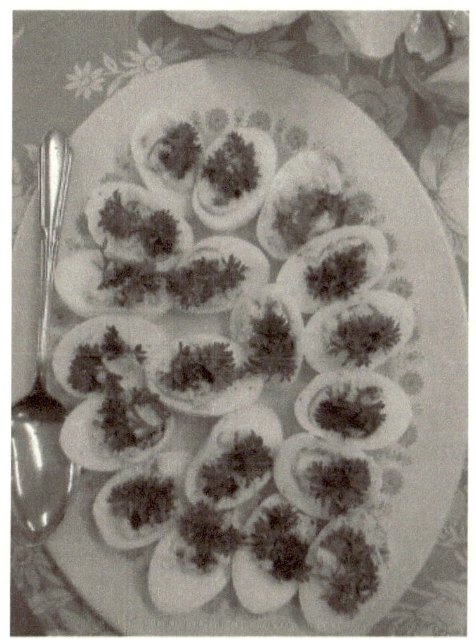

This dish is taken cold and may seem to be more suitable for summer, but winter or summer is always very appetizing and tasty.

Ingredients:

Eggs (two eggs are usually made per guest)

Mayonnaise

Ketchup

lemon juice

French mustard

tuna (canned)

salt

peas

asparagus

ersatz caviar

First, we cook the eggs for 12 minutes (hard-boiled eggs). We peel them and divide them into two halves. We carefully extract the yolks and preserve them.

Now, we will make a pink sauce by mixing a glass of mayonnaise with three tablespoons of tomato sauce (normal or fried). Add the juice of half a lemon, a pinch of salt, and a teaspoon of French mustard (if you do not have it, do not put normal mustard, just the obvious one). Add the can of tuna in oil to the sauce mix very well.

We put the mixture in a pastry bag, and we put on each half of the egg, in the space that used to occupy the yolk. Above everything, it gets a little caviar substitute. As an accompaniment, peas are cooked with salt and allowed to cool. The cooked yolks that we have preserved are crumbled and sprinkled on the peas. A couple of eggs are served per diner, a slice of cold peas with the crumbled yolk, and two or three asparagus with a generous spoonful (or a punch of the pastry bag) of pink sauce. It must be taken cold or at room temperature. You can substitute tuna for small pieces of shrimp. As the yolk, which is the one that contains the most cholesterol, it is served as a garnish, it is not a dangerous recipe for hypertensive patients or simply for those who want to care for themselves.

CREAM OF CARROTS

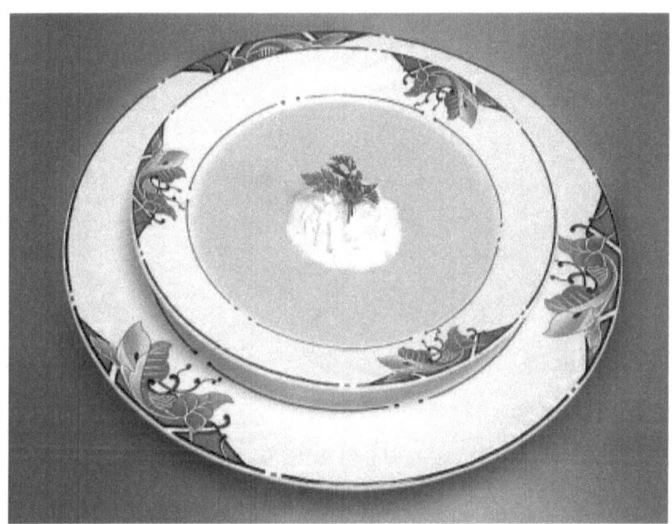

Ingredient:
4 or 5 carrots
1 onion
1 glass of milk
Grated cheese
water
Salt
In about two liters of water, we add the peeled carrots and onion, the glass of milk, and a handful of creamy grated cheese (Parmesan or similar). Boil until the carrots are soft. We pass through the blender or the paspurés rectifying salt, and it is ready to be served.

PEAS WITH HAM

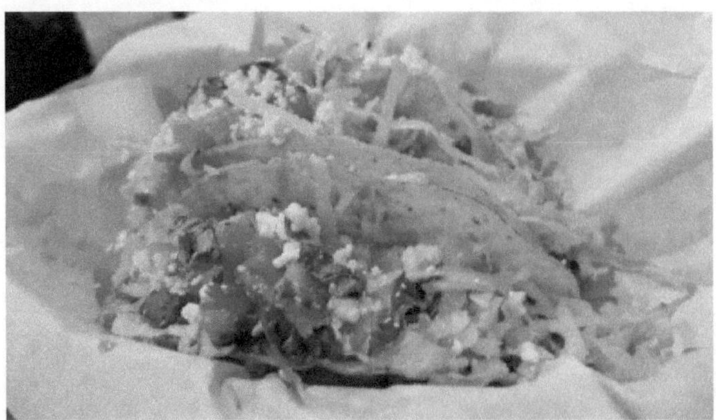

If I say that it takes 10 minutes to make the peas with ham, I probably lie since they usually have 4 leftovers.

Ingredients:

Peas according to number of diners

1 onion

1 ripe tomato

Ham

Tacos

Salt

virgin olive oil

In a pan, we fry the finely chopped onion. When it is golden, we add the tomato, also very chopped and a pinch of salt. We let the sofrito take texture.

We incorporate the ham tacos, and we give them some turns. Next, we add the peas and another pinch of salt (let's think that the ham already has enough salt by itself). We cover over low heat, and in about 3-4 minutes, they will be ready to consume.

Although I am a defender of frozen vegetables, there is a big difference between fresh and frozen peas. If you have the opportunity to make this recipe with the first, you will notice the difference. In many recipes, you will find that garlic is used in the sofrito. I don't particularly like it because it masks the delicate taste of the pea, which in conjunction with olive oil, is really impressive. But like everything in the kitchen, it goes according to taste.

SPAGHETTI WITH PRAWNS

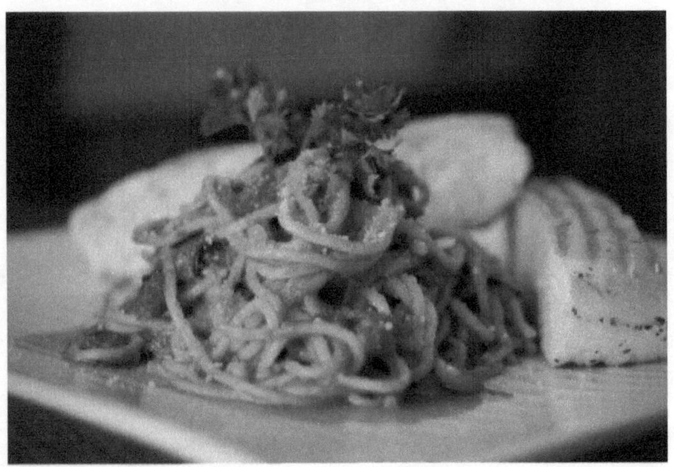

Again, a simple recipe that can be prepared in an instant.

Ingredients:

Dry or fresh spaghetti

400 grams of peeled prawns

Parsley

Oregano

3 ripe tomatoes

Garlic

1 glass of white wine or brandy/cognac

Grated cheese

Onion

Black pepper

virgin olive oil

If we start with dried spaghetti, we will take an adequate amount to the number of guests. We must think that the weight of the pasta once cooked doubles approximately the original so that 250 grams will generate 500 grams of pasta. We will boil the spaghetti in boiling water something salty according to the manufacturer's instructions, to obtain pasta al dente or soft, according to our taste. Meanwhile, in a non-stick skillet with two tablespoons of olive oil, we will have browned a garlic head and added some dried or fresh parsley, chopped well. We will throw the peeled prawns and sprinkle with oregano. Then we water with the glass of white wine or the glass of cognac and let it cook over low heat. The broth at the end of the process should be fair to keep the prawns somewhat moist.

Now we will take the tomatoes, peel them and remove the seeds to fry them in pieces in a separate pan with a little salt, very chopped onion, and black pepper. Once the pasta is cooked - between 7 and 10 minutes - we will quickly transfer it to the shrimp pan, and with a wooden spoon, we will stir it, adding some more salt. Then, add the fried tomato and after mixing again, remove from heat and consume immediately, optionally with grated cheese.

ESQUEIXAT COD

The cod esqueixat is simply the salted cod made crumbs. With it, you can make a skeleton that is basically a cod salad. It is a dish that is prepared in a few minutes.
Ingredients:
Cod crumbs
Green tomato salad
Violet onion type "figueres"
Virgin olive oil
Green and black olives
Vinegar
Salt
Desalinate the cod by soaking it in water and placing it in the fridge for about 5 hours. We will change the water at least a couple of times.

We will prepare a vinaigrette with a tablespoon of vinegar and three of olive oil. Remove the cod already desalted and put it in an absorbent paper so that there is no water left. We marinate it for an hour in the vinaigrette. Now we assemble the salad. Cut the tomatoes into slices and place them in the bottom of the plate. We incorporate the cod and the finely chopped onion on top of them (some like to make simply onion rings). We mix these last two ingredients. We put the olives on top and a little of the vinaigrette that we have used to marinate, especially to soak the tomatoes.

Optionally, you can put some salt depending on how the cod has been. It is generally not necessary since it is never perfectly desalinated.

SPINACAS A LA CATALANA

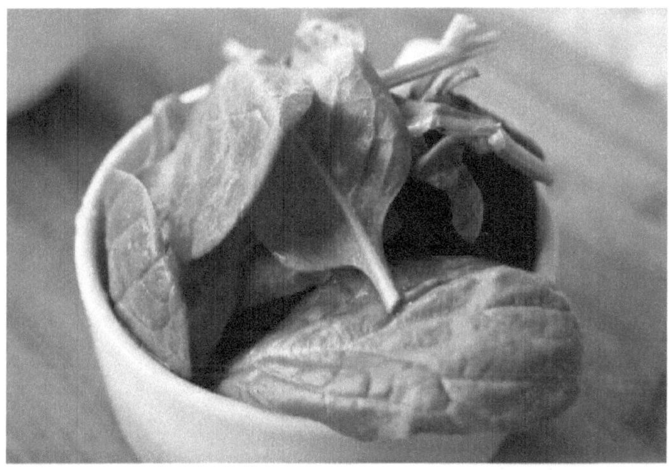

This is a very simple dish that is prepared quietly in a quarter of an hour
Ingredients:
Fresh spinach according to number of guests (300 grams for 2 people is enough)
50 grams of pine nuts
50 grams of raisins
50 grams of ham taquitos salt
virgin olive oil
If the spinach is fresh, we will have to wash them carefully because they usually contain enough soil. We will boil them in little water for about four minutes with salt. We take out and cut into pieces. In a saucepan, we pour olive oil and first fry the ham taquitos, then the raisins, and finally the pine nuts. There are people who like to sauté garlic and pass the pine nuts, although

I personally don't like it.
Then, we pour the spinach and cover. Spinach gets plenty of water, so the sauce will not burn. Simply stir occasionally and make all the ingredients scrambled. Remember to add salt and black pepper, to taste. In about 5 minutes they will be ready.

EGGS TO LA MALLORQUINA

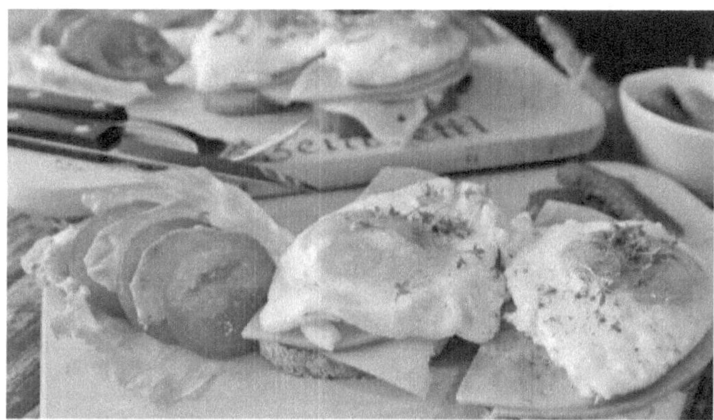

This recipe is a good excuse to use the excellent sobrasada. We will never be grateful enough to the Balearics for it.

Ingredients:

1 egg (per serving)

100 grams of sobrasada

salt

olive oil

bread

In a small clay pot (for individual use), we smear with olive oil and shell an egg. We put some salt on the yolk. We cut two slices of sobrasada and place them on the white. We heat the oven to 180 degrees and introduce the clay pot or casseroles for about 6 minutes, or long enough for the egg to solidify and make the yolk lightly (this goes to taste, we can choose that the yolk is also hard).

In a pan with olive oil, we fry two thin slices of bread and then remove the extra oil on a paper towel. The dish is served accompanied by fried bread and salt/pepper to salt and pepper to taste.

EGGS IN LEMON

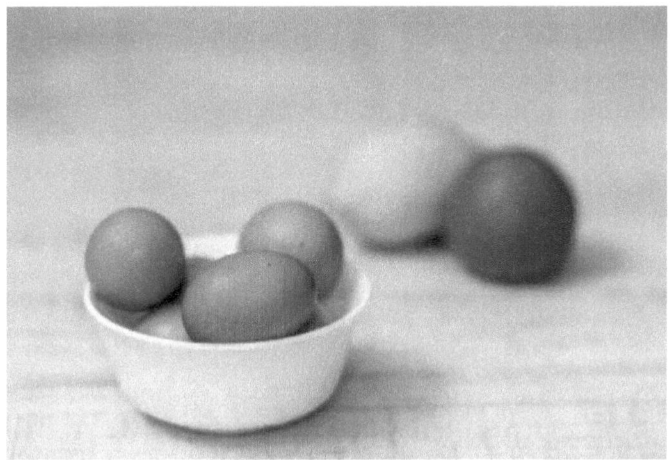

This is an extremely simple recipe.
Ingredients:
Eggs
Lemon
Virgin olive oil
Salt
Black pepper
We boil the eggs to make them hard (12 minutes). Peel and cut into sections similar in size and shape to the slice of a tangerine. We add salt and black pepper with joy. Sprinkle with virgin olive oil and lemon juice. They are served cold and are delicious.

BREAK CAULIFLOWER

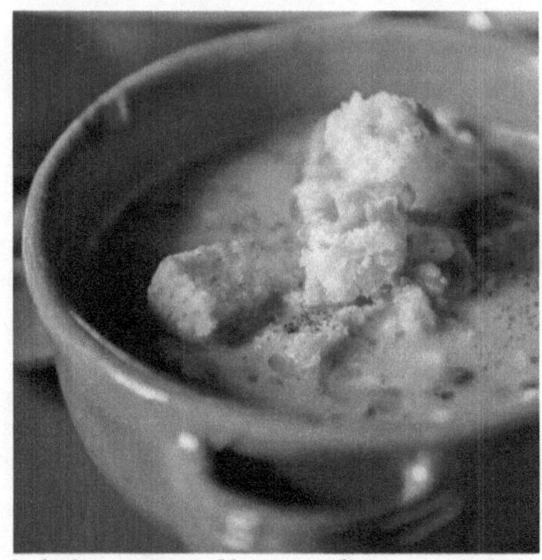

This recipe, which is generally used as an accompaniment, is a real surprise on the palate and a good way to show children that vegetables do not always have to be cooked.

Ingredients:

one cauliflower

one egg flour

water

salt

olive oil

We divide the cauliflower into small branches. In a deep bowl, beat an egg and add wheat flour and salt. To clarify the mixture, we incorporate water so that it has a consistency between liquid and paste. Ideally, we submerge the cauliflower branches and remain completely impregnated (which would not happen if it was only done with eggs or flouring first and covering with eggs later).

Shake the branch to remove the rebozo leftover and immediately put it in a deep pan with plenty of hot oil. Ideally, the branch "float" and fry quickly with many bubbles. Let's think that vegetables will be made quickly if they are small. If we make them too big, we will have to keep them longer, the batter will burn, and there won't be too much good left.

If we have problems with the size of the branches or simply because we want to make them large, we must boil them beforehand to leave them "al dente." Then we will drain them well so that the oil does not jump. If we boil them too much, they will fall apart when fried.

It is a very tasty accompaniment for meats.

BREAD SOUP

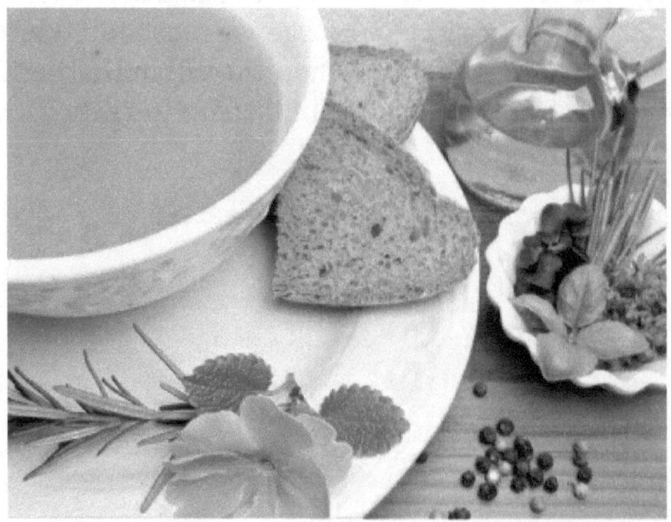

This is the soup that my family has been making for many years. It is cheap and simple to do, apart from being really good.

Ingredients:

1 liter of water

Bread (3 or 4 slices)

2 cloves of garlic

1 egg

salt

virgin olive oil

We can make this soup with hard bread or tender but fried bread. Personally, I prefer hard bread.

In a frying pan, we fry the two garlic cloves in a little oil. We preserve Heat the water until it starts to boil. Then we incorporate the hard bread and the oil with the two garlic. We stir to make the bread soften. It makes the task easier to use a rod blender so that the bread is completely undone. When we have achieved this, we will shell an egg and throw it as is in the soup. We will remove to get it to fall apart and set. We rectify salt, and it is ready to consume.

It is also possible to add some cheese on the surface and slightly gratin in the oven.

BEANS

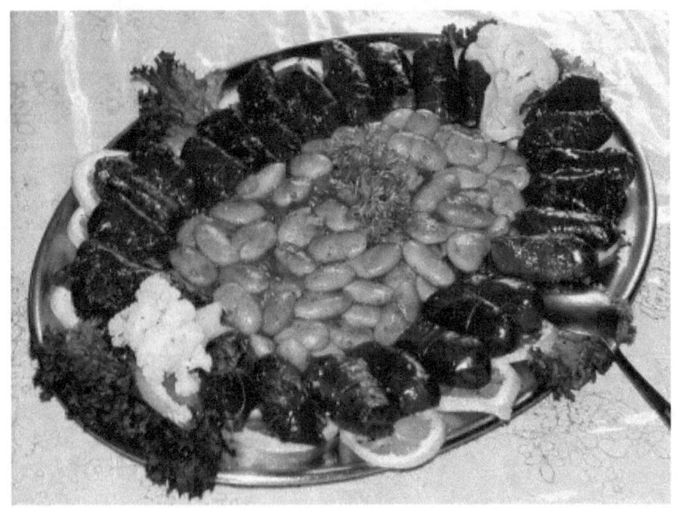

Ingredients:
½ kg of leek tender beans
1 glass of white wine (or a glass of vegetable stock)
black salt
botifarra
virgin olive oil

In a medium-sized pan with two tablespoons of olive oil pour the beans, the sliced leek, the glass of white wine, the black botifarra, and the salt. Cover the bowl and simmer. Occasionally lift and remove, ensuring that beans are not burned. If so and still hard, add a little more wine, vegetable broth, or water. The result should be that of green beans, bright and whole, soft and without any trace of broth.

PURÉ DE CALABACÍN

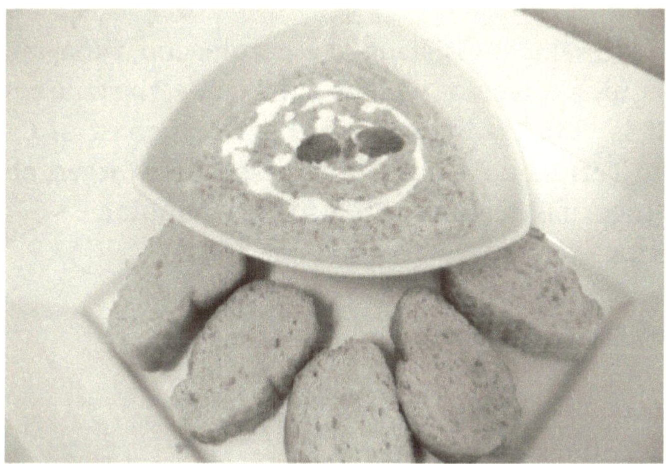

<u>I will take longer to write this recipe than I took in preparing this zucchini puree.</u>

Ingredients:
2 zucchinis
1 onion
Salt
water
olive oil

We wash the zucchini very well, and without peeling them, we remove the tips. Next, we incorporate them into 1 liter of water and a medium onion in addition to a teaspoon of salt. We boil until soft. We take out the vegetables and take them to the blender glass. We add water as thick as we want the mash and a teaspoon of virgin olive oil.

It is a very tasty recipe, easy to prepare, and especially healthy.

XATÓ

The xató is a salad consisting of escarole, cod, tuna, anchovies, and Arbequina olives, as well as Xató sauce, the true soul of the recipe. It is very traditional on the south coast of Catalonia, mainly in Tarragona, although in places like Sitges, already in the province of Barcelona, it is also very popular.

Ingredients:

Endive

Crumbled cod

Tuna

Anchovies

Arbequina olives

Ingredients for Xató Sauce:

almonds

hazelnuts

a lady *

3 cloves of garlic

3 roasted tomatoes

extra virgin olive oil

vinegar

salt and pepper

* The lady is a pepper of small size and round, which is allowed to dry and has a slightly spicy taste.

Desalinate the cod by putting it in water and letting it rest in the refrigerator for 24 hours. We will change the water every 8 hours, more or less.

For the preparation of the recipe, we first soak the escarole for a couple of hours to reduce the bitterness. We drain well and preserve it.

While we prepare the xató sauce, in a large mortar, we will incorporate the almonds and hazelnuts with a handful of salt and crush. While grinding, add the skinless lady, oil, garlic, vinegar, black pepper, roasted tomatoes, and some fried bread (the latter is not essential). Let rest.

According to the traditional method to assemble the dish, we arrange the escarole, then we throw the tuna and the cod crumbs to finish off with the anchovies, and finally, we throw the sauce. Generally, I prefer to place the escarole and pour the sauce and then work it circularly with a wooden spatula so that it soaks well. If all is well, a form of "nest" will remain, and in the center, we will incorporate the tuna, the cod, and the anchovies while the olives will be divided between the fish center and the escarole.

XATÓ

I am not one of those who claim to be one hundred percent faithful to the ways of preparation and ingredients of each recipe. I am not even with my own recipes. If I don't have lettuce today, I put escarole and so happy. The question is to analyze what is basic and what is accessory and work from that point. My opinion is that recipes are often born of improvisation and are enriched and even change completely every time someone is put on the stove to reproduce them. Notice if not in the Fideuà, a dish with its own personality that was born when embarked sailors wanted to prepare rice and realized that they had precisely forgotten the rice. It occurred to someone to put noodles instead of rice and ... voilà, a wonderful mistake.

For once, however, I will reproduce exactly the original niçoise salad recipe as it became known during the 19th century. Let no one pull their hair: the original does not carry lettuce or tuna, not even green beans.
Ingredients:
Artichoke hearts
Ripe tomatoes
Black olives
Raw red pepper (not scalded)
Anchovy fillets
Olive oil
Wine vinegar
Salt
pepper
"French" mustard
We boil the artichokes and extract the heart, the most tender part of it. We put them to marinate in olive oil with a touch of

vinegar and salt for at least 24 hours. If this is too cumbersome, we can use canned artichoke hearts, although I recommend marinating for a while before assembling the salad (without salt, canned foods usually carry an excess of it).

Peel the tomato and cut it into sectors. Cut the red pepper into slices. Now we can assemble the salad.

Place the artichoke hearts on the bottom of the plate and mix with the tomato and red pepper. We incorporate a good handful of black olives and salt and pepper. Now we will build a vinaigrette with three tablespoons of virgin olive oil, one of wine vinegar, and a tablespoon of French mustard. French mustard is very different from what we usually consume in Spain - it is strong, nasal - but easy to get. In France, they serve it with any dressing next to the vinegar and oil. If you cannot get it, it is better not to put the usual mustard because it detracts the vinaigrette, leave only the oil and vinegar. We will bathe the salad. Above all the set, we will have the anchovy fillets ... and voila.

Of course, there are extras that for many, are common in the niçoise, but it should be clarified that they are added that have nothing to do with the original recipe. For example, instead of artichokes, they use cooked green beans of the round type. Then they add tuna in olive oil, hard-boiled egg, and capers. And also, lettuce. After all, it is a salad, the kingdom of anarchy.

GRILLED PRAWNS

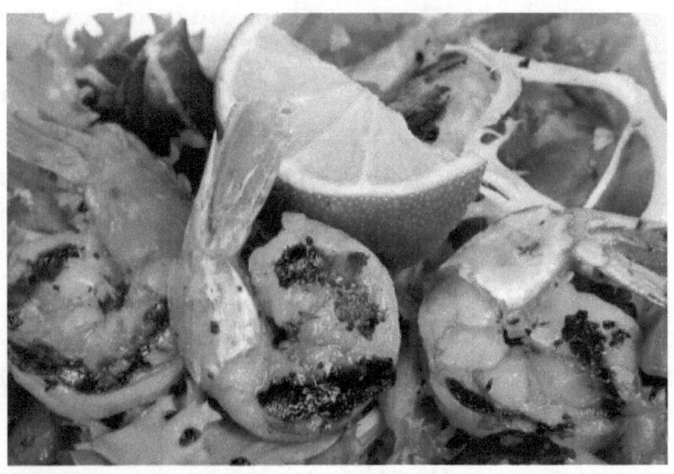

Ingredients:
4/6 large prawns (depending on the number of guests)
coarse sea salt
chopped parsley and garlic
The coarse sea salt is put on a pan for grilling and heated strongly. Prawns are deposited with a little chopped parsley and garlic. The prawns are put on a couple of minutes on each side, and they are ready to eat.

QUICK ESCALIVEDA

The escalivada is a very typical dish of Catalan cuisine that consists of roasting eggplants, ripe tomatoes, red peppers, and onion to embers of the embers and then peeling them, removing the seeds and dressing with virgin olive oil and salt. As it is clear from the way of preparation is not the type of recipe that we can easily prepare if not quite the opposite. However, if we can give up the exquisite flavor that gives the grill to vegetables, it is possible to prepare a scalded quickly and without dirtying the kitchen by simply using the microwave.

Ingredients:

1 large onion

2 or 3 red peppers

1 eggplant

2 ripe tomatoes

We use a glass container and, if possible, a microwave resistant ceramic where we will deposit the vegetables. If this is not possible, we will cut them into longitudinal strips of the largest possible size. Otherwise, it would be very difficult to peel them. Once we have arranged the vegetables in the bowl, we will bathe them in abundant virgin olive oil. We will use the microwave at a power of 700 W for 45 minutes. You may notice that the vegetables swell during cooking. This in itself is not worrisome, but we must make sure that they do not burn, which can occur if any vegetable is exposed to the microwave without being covered with oil. In the case of the volume taken by the pile of vegetables, it is not possible for all to be bathed. We will give them a review of oil with a brush.

After the relevant 45 minutes have elapsed, we will remove the container, and under running the tap, we will cool the vegetables one by one. The skin will have cracked and separated from the meat, being easy to peel the tomatoes, peppers in addition to the eggplant. We will open the peppers and tomatoes to get all the seeds while in the eggplant, we will extract as much as we can since trying with all of them would be impossible. Cut the vegetables into thin strips, add more virgin olive oil and salt according to taste. It is a recipe that can be kept a few days in the fridge and with which you can prepare toast with anchovies, mix it with cod or simply use it as an accompaniment to meats, croquettes, etc.

STEAM MUSSELS

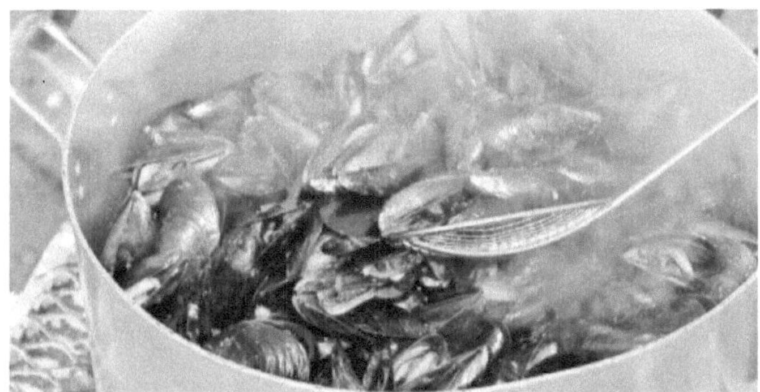

This is a really quick dish to prepare, very light and nutritious. We can use previously cooked frozen mussels or fresh mussels. Cleaning fresh mussels can take a long time, so using previously cooked mussels can save us a lot of time with similar results.

Ingredients:

1 Kg mussels with shell

Ground black pepper

Salt

1 glass of white wine

1 lemon (squeezed)

virgin olive oil

We will take a metal casserole and carefully place the mussels with the shell facing down until the bottom is covered. When this happens, we will squirt virgin olive oil and some white wine, making sure that each mussel stores some of these liquids in its shell. Then sprinkle with ground pepper. So, you proceed with the second layer of mussels and so on. Once we complete the kilo of mussels, we will put them on the fire with the covered casserole and keep them that way until the meat changes slightly in color but without hardening.

When this happens, there will be very little liquid left inside each shell. We will let them cool by bathing them then in lemon juice, although we will serve them with a broken lemon and a black pepper pinwheel so that each diner adapts it to their taste. It is a recipe that can be taken as a tapa or directly as a first course.

POTATOES WITH PEPPERS

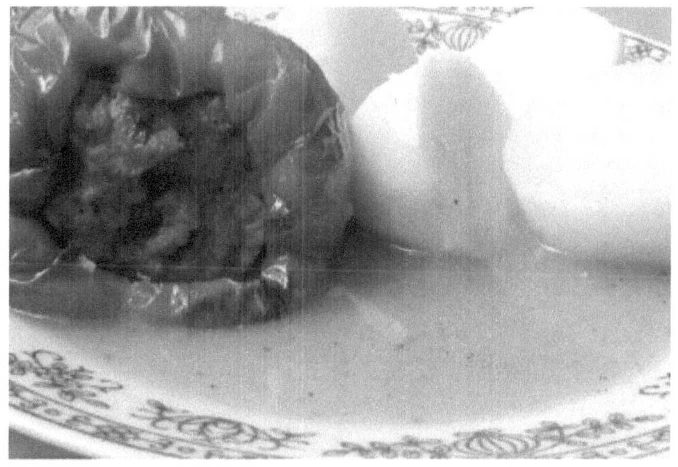

This is a simple dish that can be prepared in less than half an hour.

Ingredients:

4 or 5 medium potatoes

1 green pepper

virgin olive oil

salt

We simmer a medium nonstick skillet with virgin olive oil. We cut a green pepper into strips and fry it. Without taking it out of the pan, we throw the potatoes cut into small cubes or slices and a spoonful of salt. Over low heat, cover the pan and let it cook, stirring occasionally.

The end result will be between cooked and fried potatoes with a pleasant green pepper flavor.

COLD TUNA CAKE

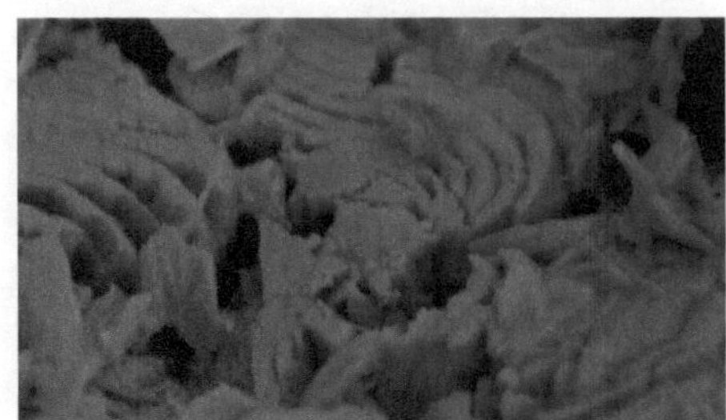

The tuna cake requires a short preparation, but consumption should be done within 24 hours so that the bread perfectly acquires the shape of the mold.

Ingredients:

1 large crusty bread without crust

1 can of tuna in olive or sunflower oil

5 ripe tomatoes

1 lettuce

1 can of red pepper or scalloped pepper

1 variant pot

1 pot of mayonnaise

boneless olives

cheese

A round or rectangular disposable pastry mold is also needed.

We take the mold and fill the bottom with the bread as a "mosaic," that is, cutting what is leftover so that it occupies all the space without mounting the pieces between them and making the round or rectangular shape as exact as possible.

We will take the tomatoes, peel them and take out the seeds and then pass them through the blender. The resulting juice will be mixed with the crumbled tuna, and with a spoon, we will spread it on the first layer of bread. We will add some salt (canned tuna usually takes it, so we will monitor the amount we will dispense).

Next, we will assemble the second layer of bread and again spread the surface with the tomato and tuna mixture. We will proceed successively until the last layer of the bread reaches the edge of the mold. When this happens, we will cut various cheese sheets to cover the bread and put it in the oven for a minute, just gratin, so that the layer of cheese is melted and of consistency to what will be the bottom once we unmold it.

We will put it in the refrigerator protected with a transparent film until the next day. We will unmold the cake with caution one hour before the meal. We will cover the entire surface with mayonnaise that we will extend with the help of a spatula or a wide knife. We will decorate the cake with olives, variants, and strips of red pepper. Finally, we will cut the lettuce into very small pieces that we will spread throughout the surface of the cake. Naturally, the way to decorate it and even the ingredients depend on the taste of each one.

This is a very simple recipe to prepare, and the result is a very delicate cake.

GARBANZOS AL WINE

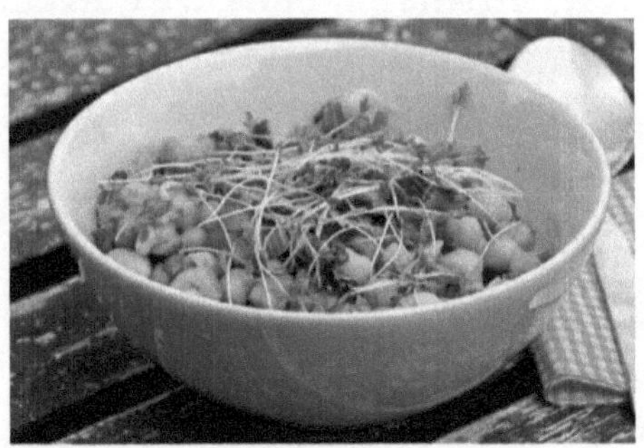

This dish hardly requires a few minutes of preparation and has a very peculiar flavor.

Ingredients:

400 grams of cooked chickpeas

2 ripe tomatoes

1 glass of white wine

1 small onion

oregano

salt

olive oil

Cut the onion into very small pieces and fry it in a pan with four tablespoons of virgin olive oil. Peel the tomatoes and remove the seeds. We cut them into small pieces and put them in the pan to avoid burning the onion. We put a pinch of salt.

Every time the sofrito has taken texture, we throw the chickpeas and some oregano. When they begin to lightly toast, we add the glass of white wine, stir and let it simmer to evaporate.

The flavor of fried-boiled chickpea with white wine is really very special; it would almost be said that "spicy."

SOUP / FISH BRACKET

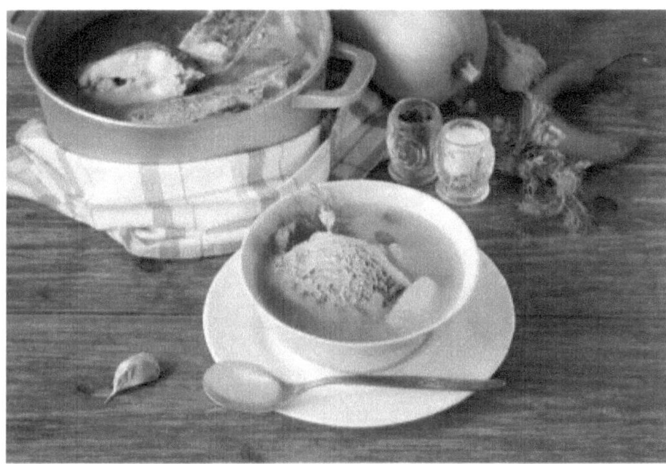

Fish broth can be used to make soups or to use in certain recipes to replace water, such as paella.

The raw material that we will use to make the broth will depend on the use that we will give it. If, for example, we want to make seafood rice, we have probably bought prawns, mussels, cuttlefish, crayfish, etc. It will not be difficult for us to remove some pieces - even if they are only the shrimp heads - and add some rockfish to complete the flavor.

Ingredients:

Prawn heads, shellless mussels, cuttlefish, rockfish, etc.

Salt

water (if possible bottled or filtered tap to reduce impurities).

We put a casserole on the fire with a liter of water and all the ingredients. Let cook for about half an hour and filter the result to prevent meat or bones from passing into the broth.

If we want to make a soup, we will make a stir-fried onion, tomato, and garlic. Then we will add the broth and some pieces of whole sea fruits such as peeled prawns, clams with shell and also if we want, a tablespoon of rice. Let it boil until the rice is soft. You can also add pasta such as noodles instead of rice. Stir-fried tomato can make some foam on the surface. This is normal, but if we want a transparent soup, we must remove the foam with a spoon.

SAMFAINE

The samfaine, like the scalded, can be an independent dish, but its use as a garnish is generally more widespread. It usually marries well with meats, chicken, croquettes, etc.

Ingredients:

8 ripe tomatoes

1 eggplant

1 big green pepper

1 small red pepper

1 zucchini

1 onion

salt

virgin olive oil

Chop the onion as if we were going to make a sauce. Brown and add then and in order, chopped but not in excess, red and green pepper, eggplant, and finally zucchini. Pepper seeds should be removed, but it is not necessary to remove the skin from the eggplant or zucchini. We will remove the ingredients, so they fry a little and release the water (it will help to add a teaspoon of salt). Finally, we will add the very chopped tomatoes, without skin, without seeds, and without the central heart if it is white. Cover the casserole and let cook until the tomato has melted and the mixture has thickened. From time to time, we will rectify the amount of salt required.

Of all the ingredients, we can only do without the red pepper since the eggplant, zucchini, and green pepper are what give personality to the samfaina.

MUSSELS WITH SPICY SAUCE

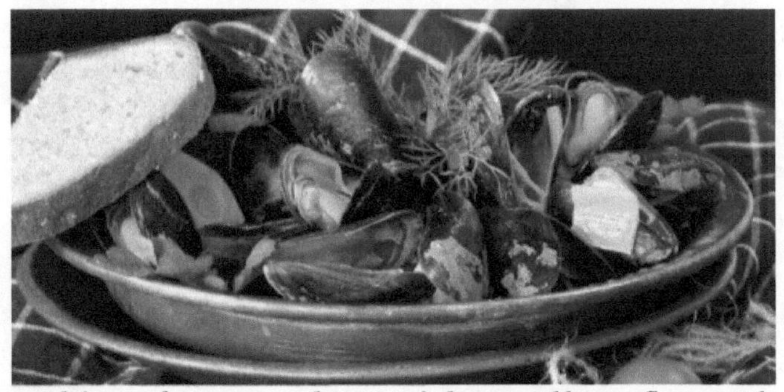

The mussel is a cheap product with excellent flavor that gives rise to many recipes.

Ingredients:

1 or 2 chopped (with bread, pine nuts, almonds, and hazelnuts)

4 ripe tomatoes

1 bottle of white wine

hard bread

water

salt

black pepper powder

virgin olive oil

1 clove of garlic

1 grain of black pepper

In a deep pot - the glass of the blender can serve us - we will pour a glass of white wine, the four ripe tomatoes without skin or seeds, the garlic clove, the salt, the chopped and the black peppercorn. We will beat until you get a uniform sauce.

We will pour the contents into a pan with two tablespoons of virgin olive oil and fry the tomato.

In the same glass where we have crushed the tomato, we will put two slices of hard bread and two glasses of water. When they have softened, we will pass them through the mixer with only two or three touches; it should not be excessively fine.

When the wine in the mixture has evaporated, we will add the bread with water and mix.

We will add the mussels with shell and washed by pouring black pepper powder on the whole (they must be spicy, so it should be generous). Let it cook for about ten minutes unless we see that the sauce dries. If this happens, we will move away from the fire.

PURE POTATOES

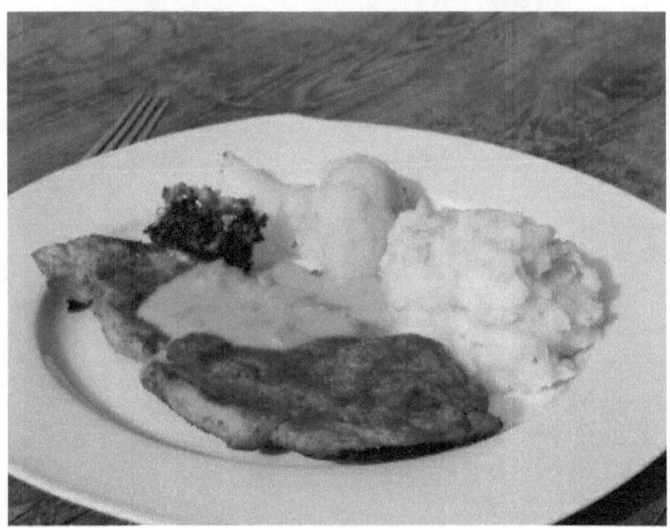

Ingredients:
3/4 medium potatoes
2 tablespoons milk
salt

Boil whole and peeled potatoes in plenty of water. When we set a fork, and it sinks easily, we will remove them to place them in the blender glass together with half a glass of cooking water, the two tablespoons of milk, and the salt. We pass it all through the blender or the pasapuré, and it will be ready to consume.

PASTA SALAD

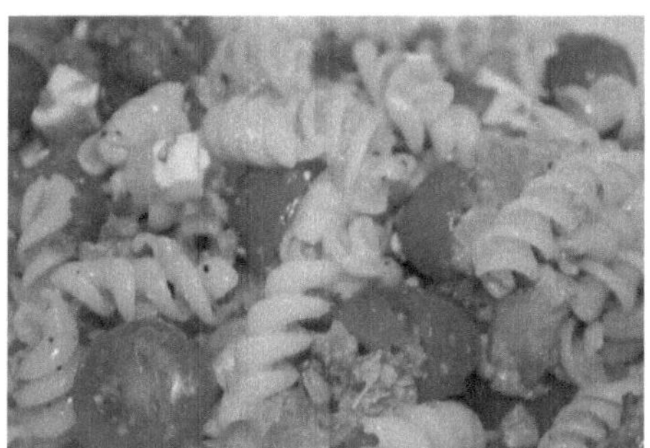

This is a typical summer dish very easy to prepare.
Ingredients:
250 grams spiral pasta with spinach and carrots
1 can of tuna
stuffed olives wide or red pepper
50 grams of arugula variants
cherry tomatoes
feta cheese
salt
oil
vinegar
mayonnaise
We boil the pasta according to the manufacturer's instructions with a teaspoon of salt. Once cooked, we separate from the cooking water and let cool but never under the stream of the tap. We add a little virgin olive oil so that it does not stick.

When the pasta has cooled, we will add the crumbled tuna, olives, variants, cherry tomatoes, and arugula and mix. If you want to give a different touch to the salad instead of variants and tuna, we will use cherry tomatoes, olives, arugula, and un-made feta cheese (without tuna or variants).

Then we will dress lightly since it will be the diner who makes the final touch on his salad. We will add salt and oil, leaving it optionally seasoned with vinegar or mayonnaise. It is conveni-ent to place it in the fridge if the maximum freshness is desired.

MACARONI WITH MEAT SAUCE

Ingredients:
400 grams of macaroni
8 ripe tomatoes
parsley
oregano
250 grams of grated minced beef
two tablespoons of milk
black pepper
salt

Boil the macaroni in plenty of water and salt according to the manufacturer's instructions. Peel and peel the tomatoes to fry them in a pan with olive oil and make a sauce. In a large skillet, we fry the meat in olive oil by adding oregano, parsley salt, and ground black pepper. Mix with the tomato sauce and work. When the sauce has acquired consistency and is homogeneous, we will pour in it the macaroni stirring so that they are well wrapped. Add the milk and let it cook together for a couple of minutes. They can be served as is or sprinkled with grated cheese and gratin.

TEMPERED SALAD

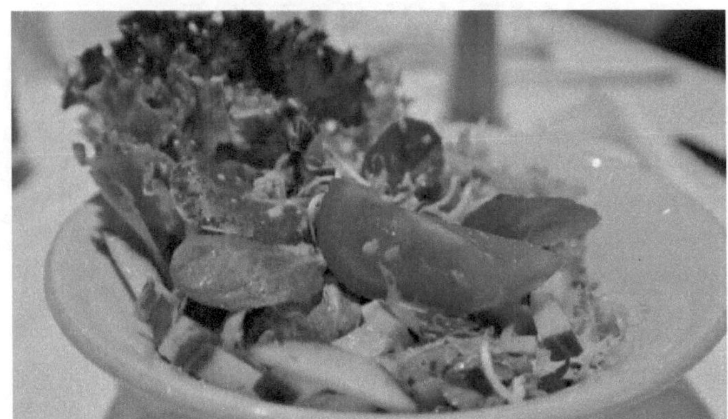

Ingredients:
1 Onion
Escarole or lettuce
olives
½ Kg of mushrooms (if possible, use fresh)
virgin olive oil
salt vinegar

We make a green salad to our liking with onion, endive, and olives. In a pan with a tablespoon of olive oil, we will place the mushrooms that we have previously washed and removed the foot. We must make the bulging part of the hat touch the pan so that where the foot was before it is facing up. This is important because heating the mushroom gives off the oil that we will collect in this improvised "bowl."

Once they are hot and with the bowl on the obverse of the hat full of natural mushroom oil, we will take them carefully and pour this oil into a ladle that we will use to spray the salad. The mushroom body will be used to crown the salad on a central mound.

VEGETABLES

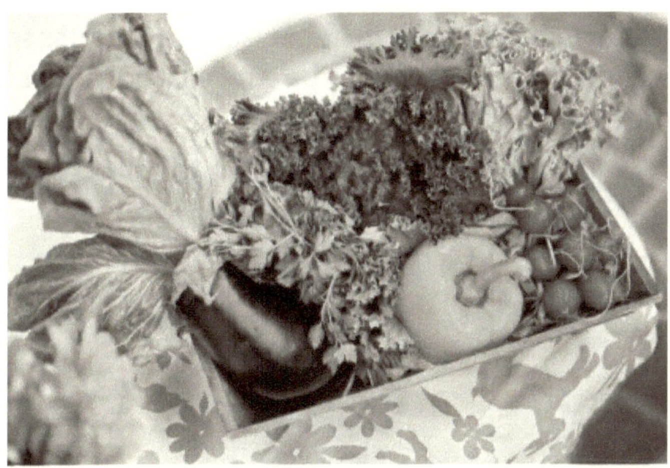

The vegetable can be a first course or an accompaniment. It can be served grilled, sautéed, or cooked. The vegetable is very important in the diet as a provider of fiber and vitamins, especially if we cook it with due respect for its beneficial components. Cook the vegetable for two hours. Of course, it will leave it soft, but all the vitamins will have died along the way.

If we boil the vegetable in water, part of its components will pass into it, so it should be boiled just as much as possible with water (obviously, the vegetable does not have to be rehydrated like pasta). Whenever possible, we will boil the whole vegetable without chopping even if we lengthen the cooking time. If we usually add potato to give more consistency to the dish, it would be preferable to boil it separately and whole since it requires more water - for a simple necessity of its size - and the cooking time is longer in general.

The best way to prepare a vegetable is steamed. For steaming, a type of bottomless casserole with a rack that is mounted on another vessel with boiling water is enough. The steam that flows through the upper saucepan perfectly cooking any type of vegetable. It is certainly the healthiest method of cooking, but the flavor of the vegetable is complete, which is why it is not usually well received by children.

The choice of one type or another of fresh vegetables should be made according to the season to be sure that it has the optimal conditions.

For example, artichokes and spinach are winter products, while cucumbers are mainly summer products.

BERENJENA, ALCACHOFA, AND CALABACÍN FRITOS

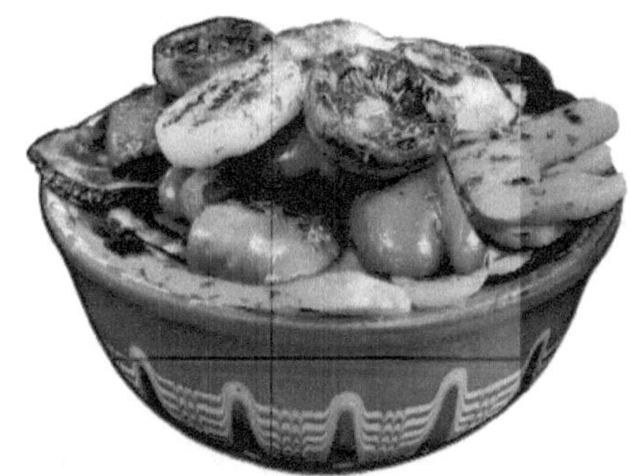

They are generally used as an accompaniment to meats.
Ingredients:
Artichoke, eggplant, and zucchini
1 egg
biscuit flour
salt
virgin olive oil
Cut the eggplant, artichoke, and sliced zucchini without removing the skin. They are salted and soaked in the beaten egg. Then they cover well with cookie flour. Quickly fry in plenty of hot olive oil.

GROUND BEANS WITH POTATOES

Ingredients:
1 potato or half potato per diner
2 or 3 flat green beans per diner
1 small onion
salt
water
We boil the diced green beans with the onion (this is optional, it just softens the flavor) in little water. After a few minutes, we add the potato cut into pieces and cover.

RUSSIAN SALAD

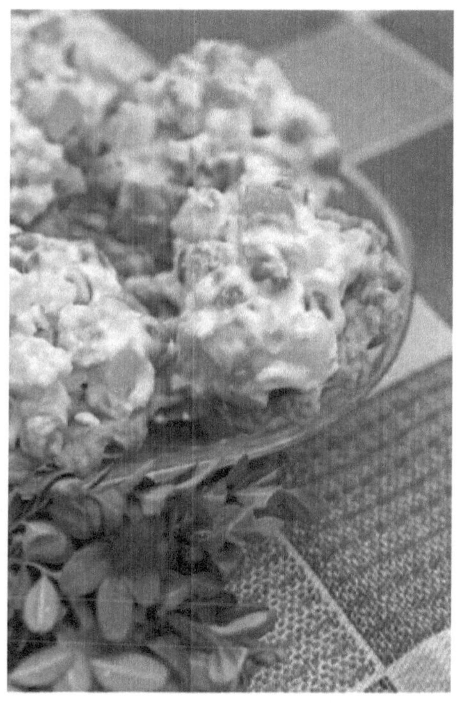

Ingredients:
potato
round green bean
peas
variants
salchichón
canned tuna
red pepper scalded
2 hard-boiled eggs
olive oil
mayonnaise
We cut the potato into small tacos and boiled. We do the same

with round green beans and peas. Let cool and preserve (without going through the cold tap water). We should have two hard-boiled eggs (12 minutes). Take them, peel, and cut into sections.

When the ingredients are cold, mix with the sliced sausage, the tuna in olive oil, and the variants. Add salt and oil and garnish with red pepper. We leave the addition of more or less amount of mayonnaise to the diner's taste.

WHITE WINE TELLIN

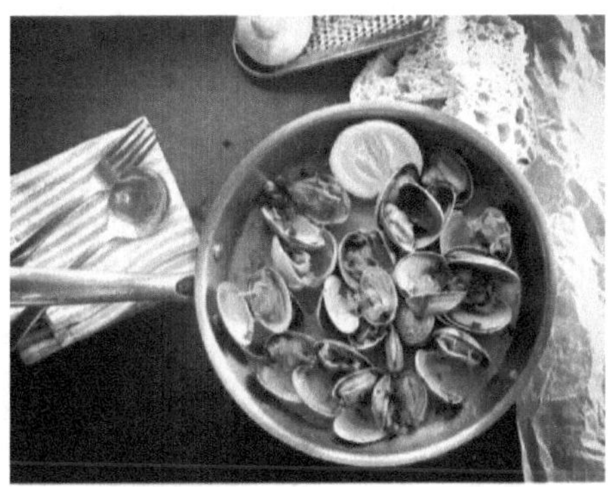

Ingredients:
400 grams of tellinas
garlic
salt
virgin olive oil
1 glass of white wine
chopped parsley

We wash and let the tellinas submerge in tap water to clean them of sand.

In a large skillet, we pour two tablespoons of virgin olive oil and heat. We pour the tellinas with a glass of white wine over low heat. We cover the pan. When the tellines begin to open, we will add salt - be careful, it is easy to pass - garlic and chopped parsley.

They are served immediately after the wine has been consumed in its entirety, although if we want them undercooked, it will be enough to leave some wine. Tellines that have not been opened should be discarded.

TOMATO AND ONION SALAD

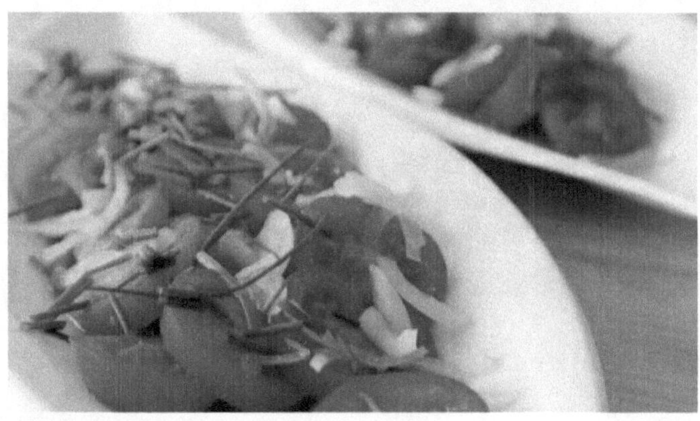

Ingredients:
4 green or ripe tomatoes (to taste)
purple onion ("Figueres" type)
cucumber
black olives

virgin olive oil
salt
vinegar
Cut the onion into rings and distribute it by a wide source. Then we add the sliced peeled cucumber and add the tomato in the same way (if it is ripe, we will remove the skin). We will incorporate virgin olive oil abundantly, olives, salt, and vinegar to taste. Wait a few minutes before serving the salad so that the onion soaks its oil flavor.

ROASTED POTATOES

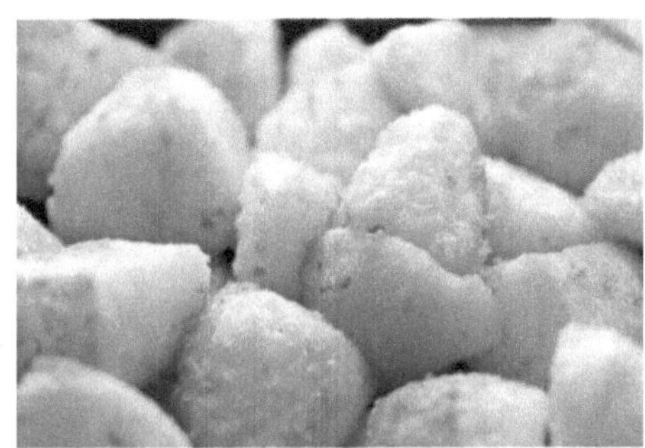

Ingredients:
Large size "mona lisa" type potatoes
salt
Ground black pepper
Virgin olive oil
We wash the potatoes well in running water. Cut the unpeeled potatoes in half throughout their length. With the help of a knife, we mark the surface of the potato with a lattice-type "three in a row" or similar, if possible, a little deep. We put salt and black pepper on all sides of each half of the potato, taking special care that they touch the area not covered by the skin. We use an oven-resistant dish that allows us to put the potatoes with the bare face-up and can be kept that way. We spray with virgin olive oil and connect the gratin. The potatoes will be ready when we stick a stick and sink, and the surface is twisted. Potatoes are served with the skin.

VINEGAR POTATOES

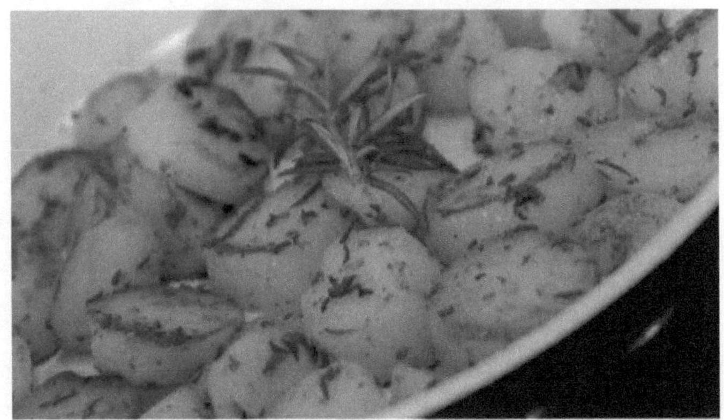

This is a simple dish that can be prepared in less than half an hour.

Ingredients:

4 or 5 medium potatoes

1 tablespoon wine vinegar virgin olive oil

salt

We simmer a medium nonstick skillet with virgin olive oil. We throw the potatoes cut into small cubes or slices and a spoonful of salt. Over low heat, cover the pan and let it cook, stirring occasionally. Halfway through cooking, we will add a tablespoon of vinegar.

The end result will be between cooked and fried potatoes with a pleasant vinegar flavor.

ANGULAS OR SURIMI

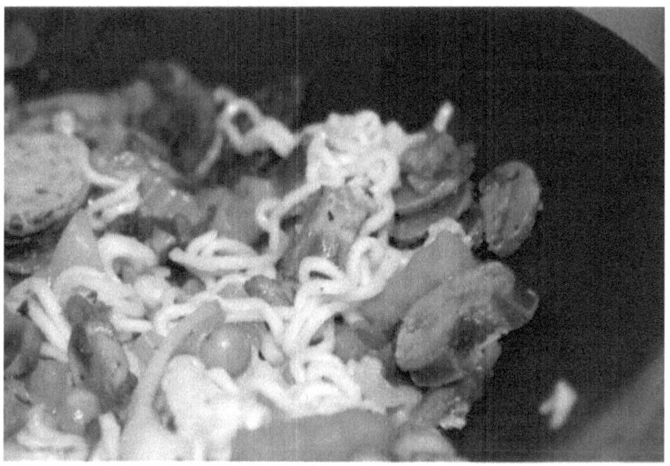

This dish can be prepared with angulas or, if we are not so lucky, with a substitute called surimi. The substitute is quite affordable and is usually acquired frozen.

Ingredients:

400 grams of surimi

1 garlic

salt

olive oil

1 bug

In a flat claypan or nonstick skillet, heat two tablespoons of virgin olive oil. We incorporate unpeeled garlic and fry over low heat. Remove the garlic after a few minutes and add the surimi with a pinch of salt and the bug. We remove, and in 2 or 3 minutes, it will be ready.

SEALED SALAD

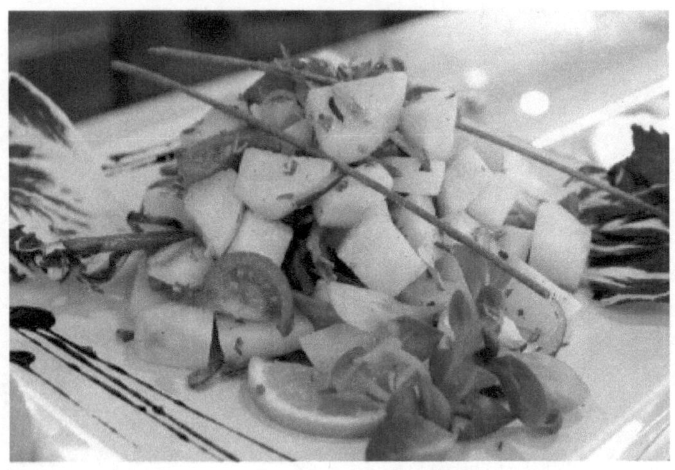

Ingredients:
250/400 grams of cooked ripe tomato
lentils
small tacos of serrano ham
virgin olive oil
salt
vinegar
We take cooked lentils and place them in a salad bowl. Peel two ripe tomatoes and shake them. We cut into small pieces. Mix with the tacos of ham. Season with salt, virgin olive oil, and vinegar, mixing thoroughly.

PUREE OF PEAS

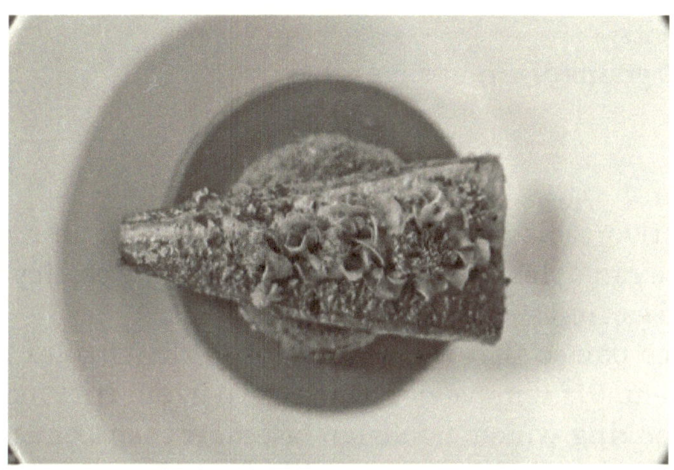

Ingredients:
2/3 medium potatoes
1 large carrot
100 grams of salt peas
We will boil the whole and peeled potatoes as well as the carrot in abundant water. Before finishing cooking, we will add the
peas. When we insert a fork, and it sinks easily in the potatoes
and the carrot, we will remove the saucepan from the fire. We
will put all the ingredients in the blender glass together with
half a glass of cooking water, and salt. We pass it all through the
blender or the pasapuré until it is very thin, and it will be ready
to consume.

GIRGOLAS

Ingredients:
200/300 grams of virgin olive oil
parsley
garlic
salt
We put two tablespoons of olive oil in a medium-sized pan. Place the gargoyles and sprinkle them with the parsley and the chopped garlic, as well as with a pinch of salt.
Cover the pan so that the own water of the girgolas helps to cook them. We remove occasionally to avoid sticking. At the end of cooking, which should not last more than 5 or 6 minutes, we will lift the lid and let the liquid evaporate.

CALÇOTS

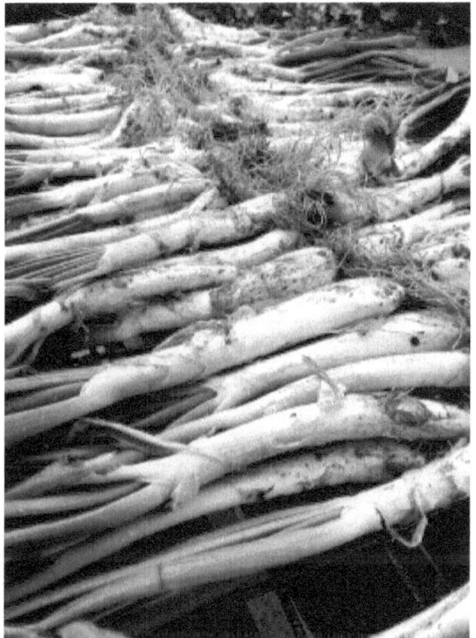

The calçot (pronounce calsót) is a typical product of Catalonia that like the snails of Lleida and the Xató of Tarragona, serves as an excuse to organize a playful-gastronomic party. Many people in the area preserve a couple of Sundays a year to eat calçots making excursions to farmhouses in the countryside where they usually constitute a single dish or strong entree of grilled meats. Due to the way of grilled preparation, it is very complicated to prepare them at home unless you have a barbecue in the garden or unless you do not mind that your neighbor hates you.

Calçot is nothing more than an onion that nevertheless has a complex elaboration process. First, the seeds are planted at the end of winter; the spring onions are transplanted. The collection is carried out in summer and attention; the bulbs are planted again in mid-September, covering them with soil as they protrude. This is done to get a completely white stem. The final result, which is obtained between winter and spring, is an elongated onion about 20 centimeters in length in its white part and a diameter of about two centimeters, with the rounded bulb typical of onions practically non-existent.

The preparation has two phases. The first is the braised-on firewood of the sarçot of the calçots. The outer layer will burn, and the inside will be soft and very tender. The second part consists of preparing a sauce in which the calçot will get wet once we have peeled the outer layer. Here, there is no label or cutlery. The calçot is taken with the hand, the outer layer is peeled, it is placed vertically in the pot that contains the sauce and thus vertical, and with the head facing the ceiling, we begin to eat it in mouths trying not to stain or stain the neighbor. In fact, the expertise - or rather, the lack of it - when eating them generates a good number of comic scenes.

The sauce used can be romesco, but more properly, salvitada is used.
Ingredients:
About 10 calçots per person for salvitada sauce:
4 ripe tomatoes
1 head of garlic
10 roasted almonds 10 roasted
hazelnuts
ñoras (2 or 3)
1 slice of crooked bread
1 bug
virgin olive oil (1 glass, more or less) vinegar
We make the tomatoes and the garlic head in the oven while we soak the ñoras and the bug.
Peel the tomatoes and the garlic head and place them in the blender bowl together with the meat that we will have scraped

off the ñoras and the bug. We add almonds, hazelnuts, and breadcrumbs. We beat it at low speed by adding the oil little by little. Finally, add the vinegar and salt.

The calçot de Valls has a designation of origin, and this town of Tarragona is the Mecca of the calçotades, although today its consumption has become widespread throughout practically the entire community.

TURKEY WITH VEGETABLES

Turkey stock is very healthy because it contains virtually no fat.

Ingredients:

300 grams of turkey for stew

1 leek celery

1 large onion

1 large carrot

4 large potatoes

200 grams of white beans

200 grams of chickpeas bottled water or filtered parsley

Twenty-four hours before starting, we will have soaked chickpeas and white beans (unless you have opted for cooked legumes).

In a large pot, we will introduce the turkey, leek, legumes, celery, onion, carrot, and the four large uncut potatoes. We will incorporate about three liters of bottled or filtered water (to remove impurities) and a sprig of parsley. Also, pour a handful of salt. We will cook for about two hours. If you have chosen the cooked legumes, you should not introduce them until about twenty minutes before the end of cooking. The process can be accelerated if you use a pressure cooker, in which case it is only possible to use dried legumes.

TIGERS (BREADED MUSSELS)

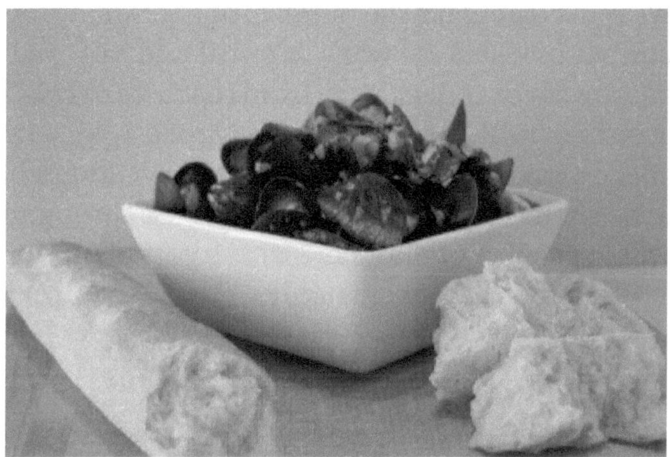

This is a typical tapas product that combines seafood cooking with the elaboration of any type of croquette.

1 kg of mussels

purple onion type "Figueres"

garlic

wheat flour

butter

1/2 liter of whole milk

virgin olive oil

egg

white wine

breadcrumbs

salt

We thoroughly wash the mussels and steam them, introducing them in a metal casserole with a glass of white wine. We remove the meat from the shells that open and preserve them. Once the segments are cold, we chop them. Now let's make the bechamel. In a saucepan, we pour oil and fry the chopped onion with a clove of garlic. When the onion is expired, we put it on very low heat. Remove the garlic and add a good spoon of butter and melting another wheat flour. We work with a spoon or some rods so that the sauce is binding. We begin to incorporate the milk little by little. When the dough is already bound, we continue adding more butter, flour, and milk without stopping the spoon. We must calculate the number of ingredients according to the number of tigers we want. We will add salt, and we will verify that the flavor moves away from the taste of raw flour and takes the taste of milk. At the end of the process, we will add the mussel pieces, mixing carefully. We separate dough balls and work on the shells to fill them. Flour and pass through a beaten egg. Then cover with cookie flour and fry in plenty of oil. Remember to rectify the bechamel salt.

TOMATO AND CUCUMBER SALAD WITH YOGURT SAUCE

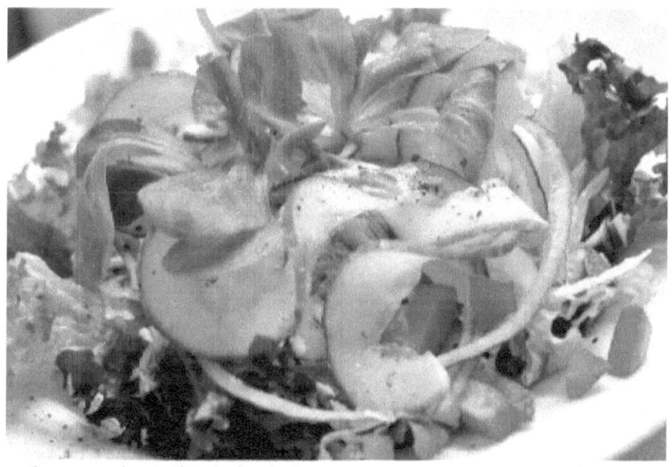

Again a "dressed" salad (with a nutritious sauce) very easy to make.

INGREDIENTS (1/2 portions):

1 cucumber

2 ripe tomatoes

1 purple onion or fresh parsley

1 unsweetened plain yogurt olive oil

vinegar

juice of 1/2 lemon

salt

ground black pepper

Peel and remove the seeds to the two tomatoes, then cut into segments like a tangerine. Chop the onion very thinly and toss it over the tomatoes. Peel the cucumber and cut it into slices, adding it to the bowl with salt, a tablespoon of olive oil and a splash of vinegar (it can be substituted with lemon). Then, mix well.

Now we are going to make the yogurt sauce. Mix the yogurt with the juice of 1/2 lemon, a pinch of salt, a tablespoon of oil, black pepper, and finely chopped parsley. It can be passed through the mixer or left as is, mixed only with the rod mixer. If we want the most liquid sauce, we can use all the juice of a lemon. We toss in the salad, and it is ready to consume.

MUSSELS IN ESCABECHE

Ingredients:
1 or 2 kg of mussels
1 glass of virgin olive oil
1 glass of wine vinegar
3 cloves of garlic
onion
bay
1 sweet pepper paprika
salt

Open the mussels to the fire with water and white wine. We take out the meat and preserve it.

In a casserole with oil, we place the garlic, the very chopped onion, the bay leaf, the clove and a teaspoon of sweet paprika and let it fry over low heat. When this cooking is underway, we add the glass of vinegar and keep it 3 more minutes. Then we see the mussels we had preserved. We leave it on the fire for about five minutes.
Let cool, put in the refrigerator and in 24 hours it will be ready for consumption. A pickle can last us a week or even longer.

LOBSTERS

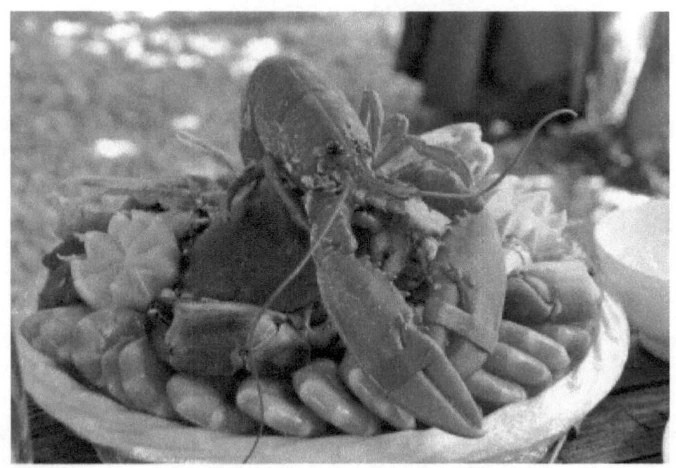

INGREDIENT:
1 Kg of prawns
olive oil
garlic
salt
oregano
1 glass of cognac (or white wine, according to taste)
In a flat clay pot with a couple of tablespoons of olive oil and a clove of garlic, we place the prawns that we have previously washed. If there are many in number, then we must arrange them in layers in the casserole. After that, we will add salt and oregano to each layer. We connect over low heat and cover the pan for about 10 minutes. Then, we pour the glass of cognac and wait for it to evaporate. When this happens, the prawns are ready to be consumed. With regard to the quality of the cognac or wine that we must use, I will only tell you that you never put a drink into a meal that you would not put in your mouth. With that, everything has been said.

NISCALO (ROVELLÓ) A LA BRASA

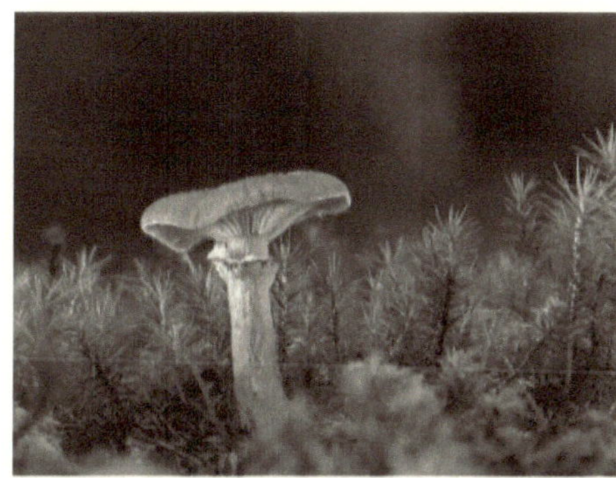

The níscalo or rovelló, as it is called in Catalonia, is a very consumed species that has not yet been cultivated. This mushroom is strongly linked to pine forests in the same way that the truffle is to holm oak forests. It has a brown-orange color, and its meat is much appreciated. It admits many preparations, but the most common are grilled and meaty.

Ingredients:

Garlic

Parsley

Olive oil

Salt

Heat the pan to grill strongly. We add a little olive oil and then the chanterelles, previously washed but without exaggeration, with the hat touching the surface. If the temperature is correct, we will make enough smoke.

Sprinkle some garlic and chopped parsley, in addition to salt. When the grill marks the hat, we will turn around, and in three minutes, it should be ready. I am of the opinion that the mushroom, and especially the chanterelle, needs very little cooking and less dressing yet, so little garlic and little parsley will be the norm. If everything has been correct, the mushroom should know and smell the pine forest when we take it to the mouth.

JUREL'S ESCABECHE

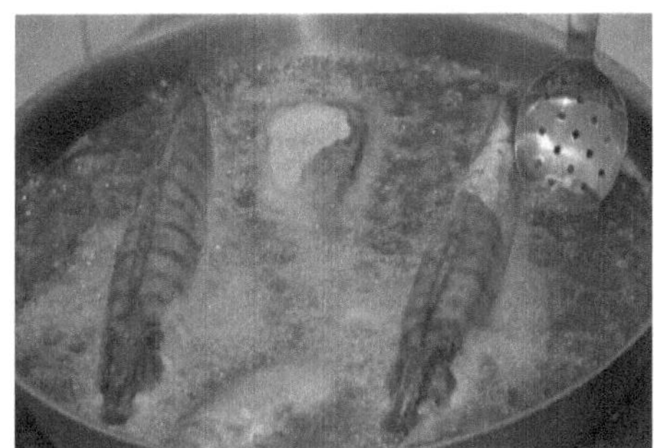

Pickling is a way to marinate vinegar previously cooked food. Vinegar is a food preservative that has been known for thousands of years. Although with fridges the marinade loses part of its usefulness, it is still carried out because it provides a very attractive taste to food. I particularly like the taste of pickled bluefish (horse mackerel, mackerel, sardine, etc.). In addition, nutritionally speaking bluefish are the cheapest and easiest source of omega-3, an essential fatty acid in the fight against cardiovascular diseases and with other very positive effects on health in general.

I have chosen horse mackerel because it is a very cheap fish and being large it is easy to eviscerate, clean, and prepare. There are many bluefish, and the process can be applied to all of them.
Ingredients:
Horse mackerel
wheat flour
1 glass of virgin olive oil
1 glass of wine vinegar
3 cloves of garlic
bay leaf
1 clove (optional)

sweet paprika (optional)
salt
We cut the head, eviscerate, and clean the horse mackerel well.
If they are large, I recommend cutting them into slices. If they
are small, we can get the supreme. Flour and salt the pieces of
fish and fry in plenty of oil. Once they are golden, we place them
in a clay pot.
In the same oil where we have fried the fish, place the garlic, bay
leaf, clove, and a teaspoon of sweet paprika and let it simmer.
Personally, I never put cloves (because I don't like the taste) or
sweet paprika because if we spend in bitter cooking. For me,
with garlic and bay leaves, it burns. When this cooking is underway, we add the glass of vinegar and keep it 3 more minutes.
Then we pour the mixture on the pieces of fish. Let cool, put in
the refrigerator and in 24 hours it will be ready for consumption. A pickle can last us a week or even longer.

CHEAP MARISCO SPLASH

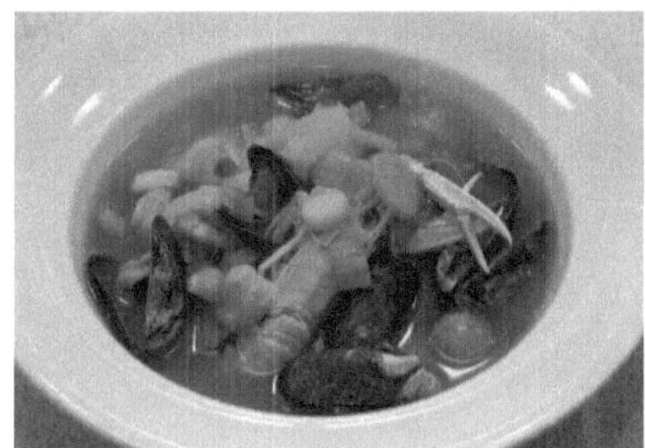

The seafood spatter can be prepared in 15 minutes and is also healthy, nutritious, and quite cheap if we do without ingredients such as prawns, prawns, etc.

Ingredients:
Mussels
Octopus
Purple onion ("Figueras" type)
Green
pepper Red pepper
Ripe tomato
salt
black pepper (optional)
olive oil
wine vinegar

Cook the octopus and mussels. The first is sliced, and the second we discard the shell. We preserve.
Chop the onion, green pepper, and red pepper very finely. Peel the tomatoes and remove the seeds, then cut into small tacos. We put all the ingredients in a bowl and salt and pepper. We make a vinaigrette with at least 3 tablespoons of wine vinegar

and half a glass of olive oil. We pour the vinaigrette in the bowl and mix. We place in the refrigerator where it must remain at least 1 hour.

XAVIER SAUCE

Xavier sauce is a type of vinaigrette. It is used in salads and to season some dishes such as cooked potatoes.
Ingredients:
olive oil
wine vinegar or apple salt
fresh parsley
egg
We take a mortar and pour the parsley with a little olive oil and salt. We work until we get a paste. We add olive oil and vinegar in a proportion of 3 to 1 (that is, if we add 3 tablespoons of virgin olive oil, we will have to put one of vinegar). We mix well. Cook an egg (12 minutes). Peel and chop as thin as possible. We add the egg to the mixture stirring well, and the sauce is ready for use. The sauce does not remain green, nor should it be homogeneous; that is, we will be able to select the ingredients. You can add shredded toast. Another way to make the sauce is to prepare the oil 24 hours before with the parsley inside so that by maceration, the flavor is transferred. Then it is no longer necessary to use additional parsley, just add vinegar and chopped hard-boiled egg.

ARTICHOKE

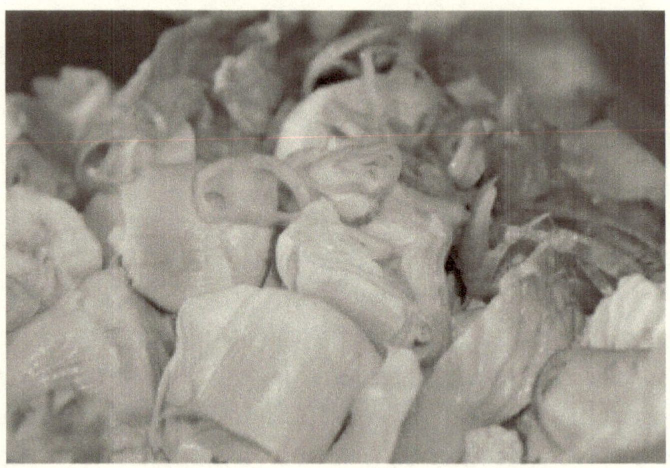

Artichoke is the flower of a plant of the same name. It is very diuretic and healthy for its beneficial effects on diabetes, cholesterol, etc. Virtually all diets include artichoke, although limiting a diet to ingestion can be harmful in the long run.

Ingredients:
2 or 3 artichokes per person olive oil
Salt

Ideally, prepare the artichokes outdoors, in the barbecue of our garden, near the pool, but if your house is 55 square meters and luckily, you can have a couple of pots in the window - exactly as I live - then the oven is a good substitute.
Artichokes are a winter product, although thanks to modern conservation techniques, we can find them almost throughout the year. In any case, I recommend eating the vegetables according to their season since the rest of the time, the quality is not

the same, and the techniques to preserve them can affect the flavor.

We take the artichokes and wash them well. We do not remove the outer leaves because, despite being hard and inedible, they will serve to protect the delicate interior.

To open the flower, we will hit the opposite end of the stem against the kitchen table. Turn the alchachofa and sprinkle salt, sprinkling with olive oil, making sure it reaches the heart. For this to happen, we must keep the artichoke with the stem down. We will use a glass tray for the oven, if possible so that we "squeeze" the artichokes and do not fall sideways. We will introduce in the oven at 180 degrees for about 30 minutes, although we will watch to take it out when the outer leaves begin to blacken.

They eat as we defoliate a flower: we ripped the leaves and eating the part closest to the heart, which is also the most tender and almost white in color. Naturally, as we move towards the center, there will be more tender and, therefore, edible parts. Sometimes we can dip the leaf in some kind of sauce such as romesco, aioli, etc.

In late winter and early spring, we can make combinations of baked artichokes and wild asparagus that are really tasty.

CABAÑIL GARLIC

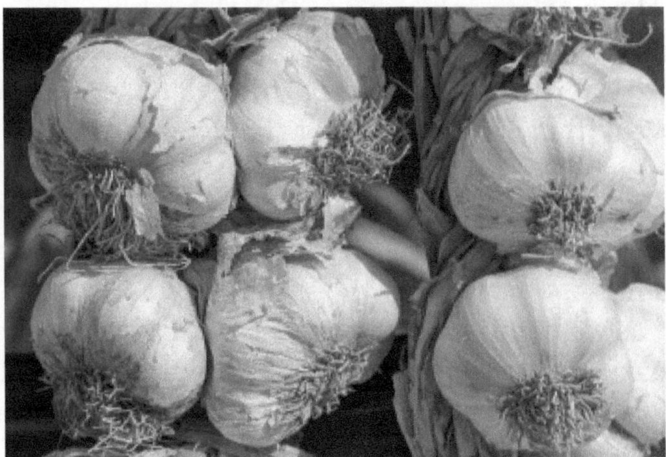

An important contribution of Murcian cuisine is the sauce called garlic cabañil that can be applied to many dishes, from simple potatoes to lamb chops through the rabbit. The simplest way to make cabañil garlic is to crush three garlic heads in the mortar by mixing them with three tablespoons of vinegar, two of water, and salt. A somewhat more elaborate form includes fried bread, almonds, and bay leaf. In any case, you should not miss vinegar and garlic, the two essential elements that define this vinaigrette. A "universal" way of applying it is to cook the base element routinely and add the garlic about ten minutes before the end of cooking to simmer the meat or the frying of the potatoes.

ALIOLI

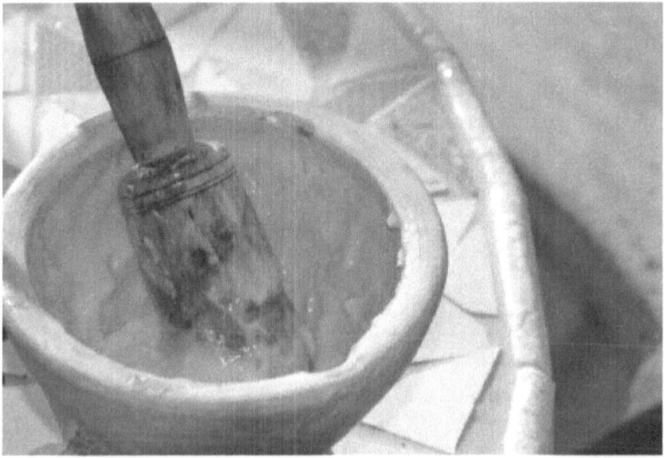

The name says it all: garlic with oil. It would be the simplest and cheapest sauce to make if it weren't for the small detail: it tends to be cut. Sometimes, to avoid this unpleasant "cut," you can start flirting with a bit of mayonnaise.
Ingredients:
4 cloves of garlic
1 glass of virgin olive oil salt
mayonnaise

In a mortar, we put the four peeled garlic cloves and a little salt. We begin to crush them to form a homogeneous paste. Now comes the hard part. Without stopping working, we pour the contents of the glass of oil little by little (I recommend using a sterile or alcuza) until the sauce is binding. If we have any - bad - previous experience, we can start with a bit of mayonnaise and then start linking oil. It will be ready when a yellowish and homogeneous sauce is left. We will know if it has been cut simply when we see that garlic paste and oil go "free." Luck and bull, because it is worth it. It is ideal to accompany grilled meats, roasted potatoes, black rice, and even fish.

CHAPTER 6 - MAINS

STRIPE WITH GREEN SAUCE

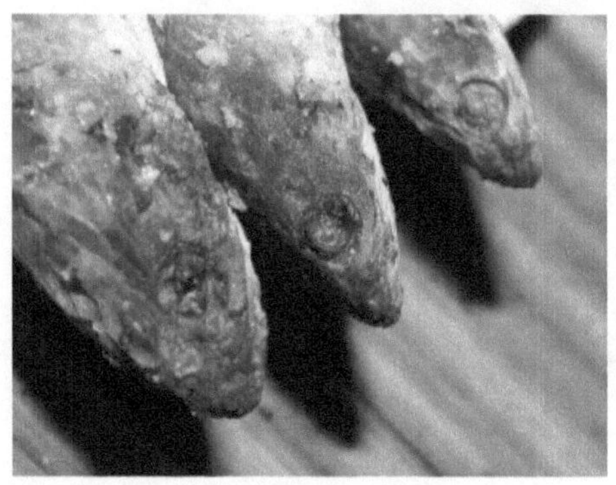

Ingredients:
4 pieces of stripe
fresh parsley
garlic
wheat flour
1 glass of wine
salt
water
virgin olive oil

We will batter the stripe pieces of flour and fry them in a pan with oil where we have previously browned garlic. We will remove them and preserve them.

In the same oil where we have fried the line, we will add a couple of tablespoons of wheat flour and work it to cook it. We will add a glass of white wine, salt, and chopped parsley and let it boil working the sauce until it takes consistency. We take the pieces of stripe and put them in the sauce so that they cook together for a couple of minutes.

LAMB WITH BEANS

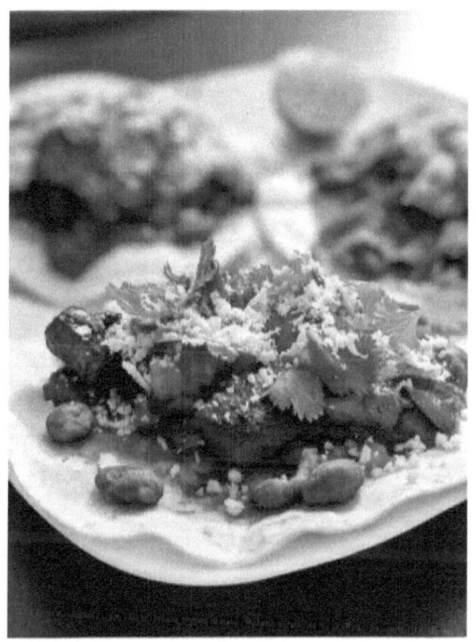

Ingredients:
5 or 6 fillets of lamb legs
onion
tomato
potatoes
100 grams of beans
leek
1 mint leaf
1 glass of wine
vegetable broth
salt
virgin olive oil
Fry the leg of lamb fillets in virgin olive oil without making them too much. In a flat casserole, we will make a fried onion

and tomato sauce. We will add the potatoes and brown them lightly. Next, we will pour a glass of white wine, a piece of leek, and the mint leaf. We will keep boiling until the wine evaporates. Once this happens, we will add vegetable broth or water, failing with beans. We will put on low heat, and we will rectify salt until the beans and potatoes are soft enough.

LENTILS

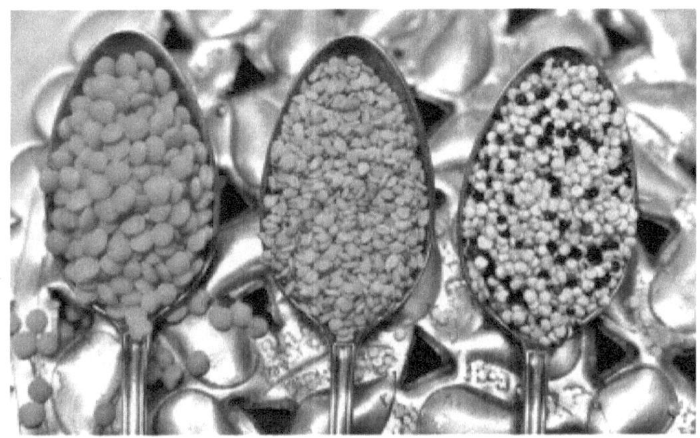

Ingredients:
400 grams of dried onion lentils
potatoes
1 bay leaf
1 ham bone
1 black pudding
1 stew sausage
We will keep the lentils dry in a bowl of water for twenty-four hours. We take a casserole with two liters of water and add a whole onion, bay leaf, ham bone, and lentils. We add salt.

Halfway through cooking, we put the potatoes, the blood sausage, and the sausage to cook. It is preferable that the potatoes are medium and are placed whole. The lentils will be ready when they are soft, as well as the potatoes. It is convenient to serve by removing the onion - or parts of it if it has been undone - and the bay leaf, basically because of the comfort of the diner. Regarding the meat that we have introduced, we can either distribute it or simply discard it.

SEPIA WITH POTATOES

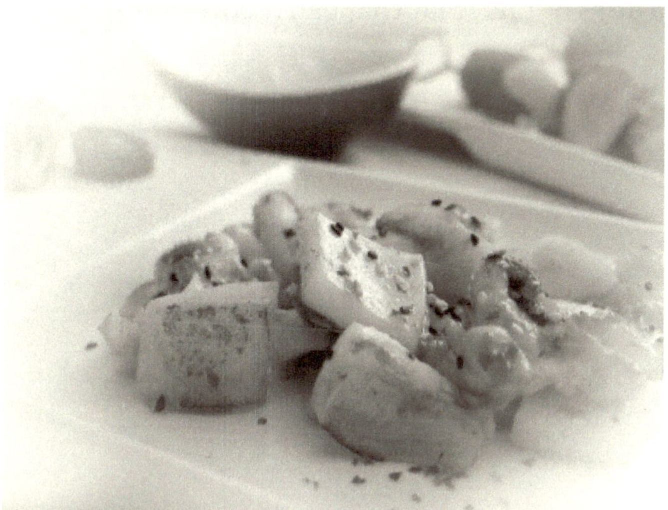

This recipe can be used as a single dish because it contains the sepia protein and all the vegetables we want to add.
Ingredients:
1 fresh or frozen sepia
4 or 5 medium potatoes
100 grams of peas or green beans
one carrot onion green pepper
two ripe salt tomatoes
virgin olive oil water
In a clay pot, we make a sauce with green pepper, tomato, grated carrot, and onion. The order of the ingredients for the sofrito will be in the order of hardness, being first the carrot, then the pepper, the onion, and finally, the tomato. Cut the cuttlefish into slices and add them to the sofrito to brown slightly. We incorporate the salt.

We cut the potatoes into small squares and place them in the casserole together with the peas. We cover the ingredients completely with water - if it has been previously heated, the cooking will be faster - and let it cook until the potatoes are soft and part of the water has evaporated. The dish is not only served with broth, but if you want, it will be preferable to crush some potatoes and return them to cooking to give consistency since the sepia does not have fat that can incorporate into the water.

RICE WITH FRIED EGG

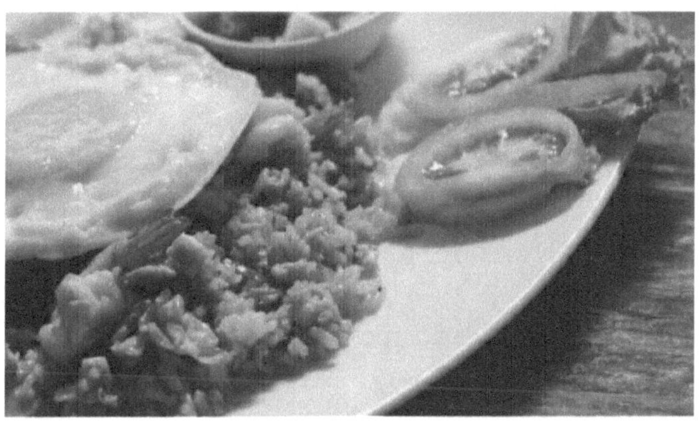

Ingredients:
200 grams of rice (a glass of grocery store, approximately)
6/8 tomatoes
eggs
salt
garlic
virgin olive oil

In a casserole with plenty of water, boil the rice with salt until it softens. Peel the tomatoes, remove the seeds and fry in oil where previously we will have lightly browned garlic. In another pan, we will put plenty of oil that we will heat over medium heat. When it is very hot, we will break an egg and being careful not to break the yolk. We will fry it.
The plate is mounted as follows: we take the rice once drained and form a crown around the plate. Then we paint on top of the crown with the tomato sauce. In the center that will be obviously empty, we carefully deposit the fried egg that each diner will season to their liking.

RICE

The base of rice is the sofrito, whatever its variant is. For chicken rice, we will use the simplest onion and tomato stir fry with a touch of garlic, while for fish rice, we will add green pepper. It should also be noted that it is possible to prepare a bowl of rice in half an hour as long as the following is taken into account:

1. we must "fry" the rice to accelerate its cooking

2. We will always use very hot water or broth every time we have to add it.

3. We will try to use the same type of rice always and, if possible, from the same supplier. Thus, we will know very well the cooking process and all its peculiarities, correctly anticipating the amount of water and salt needed. For

For getting started in the world of rice, I advise pump rice.

Although we know that it is not the way to do it, it is possible to accelerate the cooking of the rice by adding it to the sofrito and working it so that it does not stick. In addition, we will always add very hot broth.

MIXED RICE

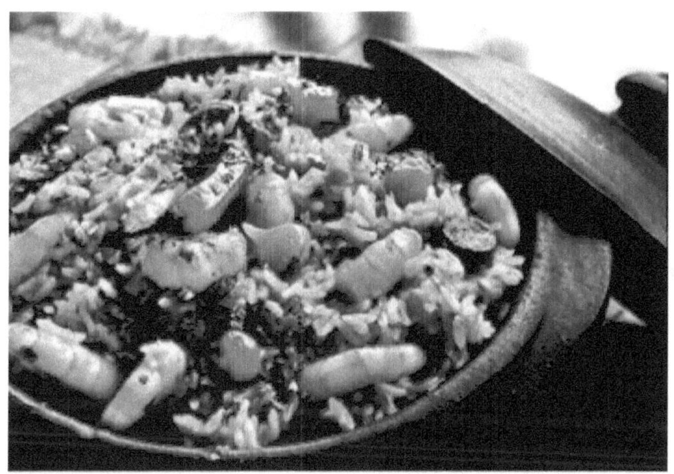

Ingredients:

onion

green pepper

1 ripe tomato

garlic

200 grams of pump-type rice (4 people) that becomes a full glass of water.

½ liter of fish stock or squid water

mussels crayfish

prawns (unpeeled)

artichokes

peas

split chicken wings

Pork ribs or salt rabbit loins

saffron or paprika virgin olive oil

If we have fish stock, we will heat it over medium heat. If we didn't have it, we could do it with some soup fish, shrimp heads, etc. And if there is no other choice, we would use water.

In a paella where we pour 2 tablespoons of olive oil and brown a garlic. Once it is golden, we will remove it to add the onion, the green pepper, and the tomato finely chopped. Now we can include some strand of saffron or a small spoonful of sweet paprika. Then we will add chicken wings and pork ribs to brown. Finally, we pour all the rice in the center to fry lightly and speed cooking. The salt should be added at the same time that we put the rice because then it would be very difficult to rectify it (the rice does not admit the salt when it is already cooked). We won't stop working and stir the mixture to prevent the rice from burning.

When it begins to brown the water, or the broth should already be boiling. The broth is poured with a soup ladle until the rice is covered with high, and it is boiled for about 15-20 minutes. We preserve a glass of broth that we will keep warm. Halfway through cooking, we will add the vegetables, other strands of saffron, and two or three minutes before putting out the fire, the crayfish, shrimp, and mussels. To know when the rice is made, we will try some grains throughout the cooking. In the beginning, there will be many hard ones to then go down the number as the cooking progresses. If we see that twenty minutes have passed and there are still many hard ones, we will add another ladle of broth, and if instead, they are all soft, we will immediately close the fire. Rice is always preferable to be a little whole before the last. That is why when the fire is extinguished, and when the broth has evaporated, we will let the stew rest for 10 minutes so that the rice, which is very greedy for water, finishes absorbing it and softens. (all this with the paella discovered) If, after ten minutes, there are still hard grains, we will cover the paella with aluminum foil and wait another time and until all the rice is homogenized.

RICE WITH COD

Ingredients:
onion
green pepper
1 ripe tomato
garlic
200 grams of pump-type rice (4 people) that becomes a full glass of water.
½ liter of fish stock or water
Salted cod crumbs or cod loin (1 per person).
artichokes
peas
salt
virgin olive oil
saffron or paprika

The day before, we desalted the cod by dipping it in water and putting it in the fridge for 24 hours. We will change the water two or three times to eliminate the extra salt. If we have fish stock, we will heat it over medium heat. If we didn't have it, we could do it with some soup fish, shrimp heads, etc. And if there is no other choice, we would use water.

In a paella where we will pour 2 tablespoons of olive oil, we will brown the garlic. Once it is golden, we will remove it to add the onion, the green pepper, and the tomato finely chopped. Now we can include some strand of saffron or a small spoonful of sweet paprika.

When the sofrito takes the body, we will add the rice to fry it slightly and accelerate the cooking. The salt should be added at the same time that we put the rice because then it would be very difficult to rectify it although we must be careful because the cod despite being desalinated is never 100%. We will not stop working and stir the mixture to prevent the rice from burning. When it begins to brown the water, or the broth should already be boiling. The broth is poured with a soup ladle until the rice is covered with high, and it is boiled for about 15-20 minutes. We preserve a glass of broth that we will keep warm in case we need to add water later. Halfway through cooking, add the cod. To know when the rice is made, we will try some grains throughout the cooking. In the beginning, there will be many hard ones to then go down the number as the cooking progresses. If we see that twenty minutes have passed and there are still many hard ones, we will add another ladle of broth, and if instead, they are all soft, we will immediately close the fire. Rice is always preferable to be a little whole before the last. That is why when the fire is extinguished when the broth has evaporated, we will let the stew rest for 10 minutes so that the rice, which is very greedy for water, finishes absorbing it and softens it. (all this with the paella discovered) If, after ten minutes, there are still hard grains, we will cover the paella with aluminum foil and wait another time until all the rice is homogenized.

ESTOFADO RABBIT

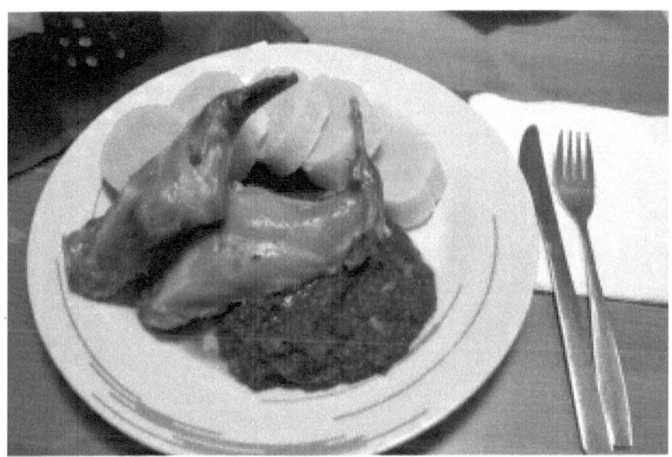

Ingredients:
½ rabbit
onion
water or vegetable broth
salt
olive oil
We will wash the rabbit and chop it by rejecting the head. Fry the parts together with the liver and preserve it. We should get a golden external appearance, although internally, it may not be completely done.

In a flat clay pot, we will make a stir-fried onion and tomato grating the liver that we have previously fried. Then add the cut potatoes and brown them in the sauce with a little salt.

Now we introduce the rabbit, the peas and the bay leaf and fill with broth or water up to 2/3 parts of the casserole, without covering the rabbit. Let cook over medium heat for half an hour,

occasionally checking the salt point and the hardness of the potatoes. If we want to give more consistency to the broth - although it is really served with very little
- We will crush a couple of pieces of potatoes and return it to the broth five minutes before finishing the preparation.

VEGETABLE RICE

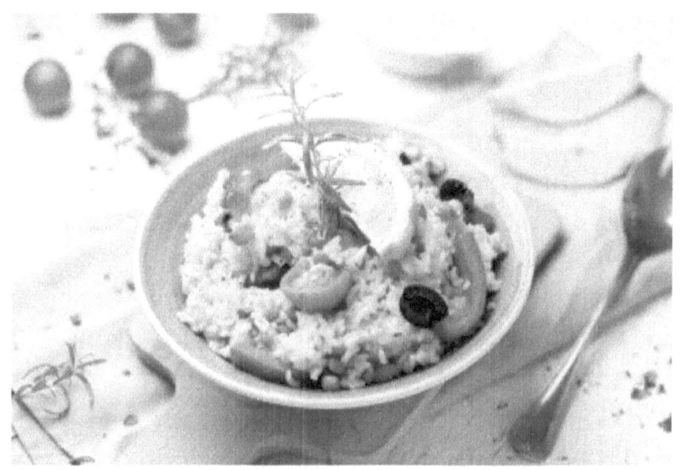

Ingredients:
onion
green
pepper red pepper
zucchini
eggplant
artichokes
peas
1 ripe tomato
garlic
200 grams of pump-type rice (4 people) that becomes a full glass of water.
½ liter of vegetable stock or saltwater
saffron or paprika
virgin olive oil
If we have vegetable broth, we will heat it over medium heat. If we did not have it, we could do it with onion, celery, leek, etc. And if there is no other choice, we would use water.

In a paella where we will pour 2 tablespoons of olive oil, we will brown the garlic. Once it is golden, we will remove it to add the onion, the green pepper, and the tomato finely chopped. Now we can include some strand of saffron or a small spoonful of sweet paprika. Next, we will add the vegetables to the sofrito in order of hardness. First, we will throw the finely chopped red pepper and then the diced zucchini and eggplant and keeping the skin. We will work the mixture to prevent burning. When the mixture comes together, we will add the rice to fry it slightly and accelerate the cooking. Salt should be added at the same time we put the rice because then it would be very difficult to rectify it. We will not stop working and stir the mixture to prevent the rice from burning. When it begins to brown, the water or broth should already be boiling. The broth is poured with a soup ladle until the rice is covered with high, and it is boiled for about 15-20 minutes. We preserve a glass of broth that we will keep warm in case we need to add water later. Halfway through cooking, add the sliced artichokes and peas. To know when the rice is made, we will try some grains throughout the cooking. In the beginning, there will be many hard ones to then go down the number as the cooking progresses. If we see that twenty minutes have passed and there are still many hard ones, we will add another ladle of broth, and if instead, they are all soft, we will immediately close the fire. Rice is always preferable to be a little whole before the last. That is why when the fire is extinguished when the broth has evaporated, we will let the stew rest for 10 minutes so that the rice, which is very greedy for water, finishes absorbing it and softens it. (all this with the paella discovered) If, after ten minutes, there are still hard grains, we will cover the paella with aluminum foil and wait another time until all the rice is homogenized.

CHICKEN WITH PINION

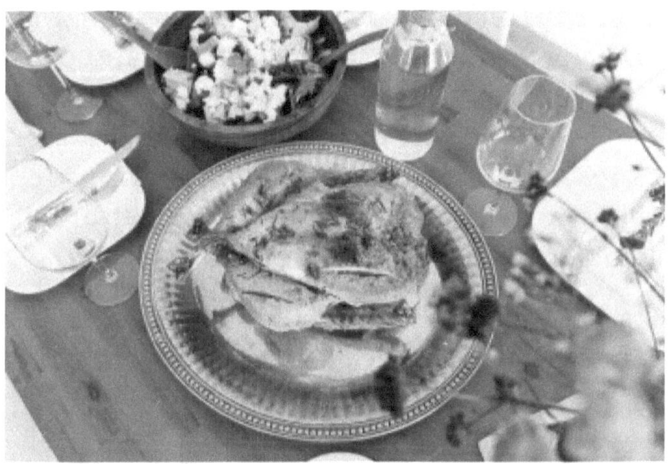

Ingredients:
4 chicken drumsticks
1 ripe tomato
4 medium potatoes
onion
50 grams of pine nuts
virgin olive oil
salt
garlic
In a flat clay pot, we heat unpeeled garlic in virgin olive oil. We will remove the garlic after a few minutes and lower the heat. Chop the onion very thinly and toss it with the peeled tomato, seeded and cut into pieces. Next, we will throw the pine nuts stirring constantly. We will cut the potatoes into medium-sized dice and brown them together with the sofrito. Potatoes should be lightly fried.

Before the pine nuts are roasted in excess, we will proceed to pour the four chicken drumsticks and fill the casserole with water up to two fingers of the edge. It does not matter if the thighs protrude because we will go around them throughout the cooking. Add the salt.

The dish will be ready in about 30 minutes. If we want to speed up the process, we can make the thighs in a pan and then add, but the taste differs. It is also not desirable to use strong fire because the meat will be too hard or well the broth will evaporate, leaving the raw thigh inside. You can use chicken or vegetable broth instead of water and, without problems, you can accelerate cooking by boiling the broth separately.

The dish is well made when the thigh is well done inside, it is very soft, and the flavor of the pine nut is predominant.

LOIN WITH TOMATO

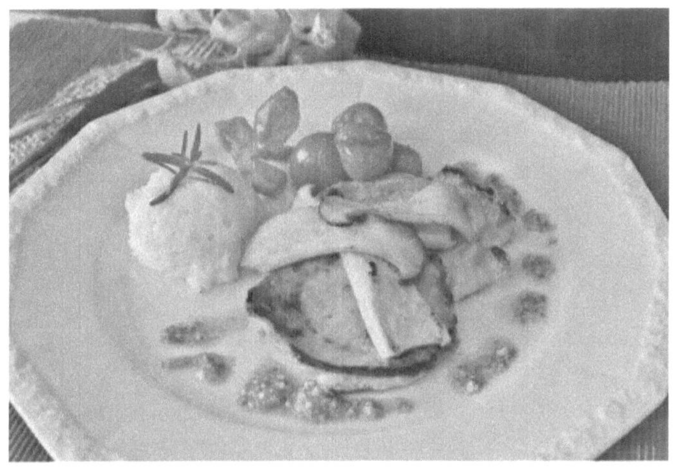

Ingredients:

400 grams of tenderloin

8 ripe tomatoes

1 can of red pepper or a scalded red pepper

virgin olive oil

ground black pepper

salt

Lightly fry the loin seasoned in olive oil. Peel the tomatoes and remove the seeds. Fry the tomato by mixing it with the red pepper and the salt. When the sauce acquires texture, we will pour it into the meat. The last 5 minutes of cooking will be done together with meat, tomatoes, and pepper. The addition of scalded pepper to tomato sauce changes the taste of it very positively.

MACARONI

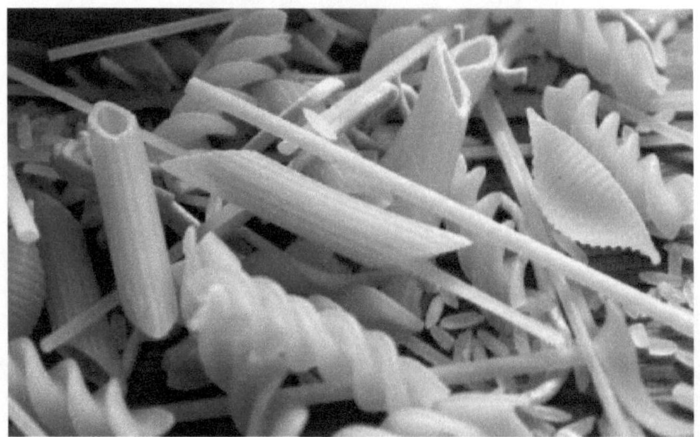

The philosophy of macaroni and broth is to add macaroni and meat to a vegetable broth base for consistency.

Ingredients:

200 grams of dried macaroni

vegetable stock (celery, carrot, leek, and onion)

potatoes

100 grams of lean meat

black pudding salt

We make vegetable stock with bottled water or filtered tap and celery, carrot, leek, and onion. We can use it at the moment or preserve it and use in various dishes.

Add the meat, a couple of whole small potatoes, and the black pudding to something more than a liter of vegetable stock. When the meat is cooked, we add the 200 grams of macaroni and boil until they are al dente or made (according to taste). We will be careful to rectify the salt as the dish is prepared.

FILLED CHICKEN

Ingredients:
1 whole and emptied chicken
200 grams of minced beef
1 hard-boiled egg
boneless white olives
pine nuts
red pepper (scalded)
salt
ground black pepper
virgin olive oil
In a pan with two tablespoons of virgin olive oil, we fry the minced meat by adding salt and ground black pepper. When it takes color, we add the pine nuts and the red pepper. In a saucepan with water, we will have made a hard-boiled egg (12 minutes) that we will peel and make pieces to incorporate into the dough of the filling.

We take the chicken and clean the interior with plenty of water. With the help of a spoon, we fill it with the mixture we have prepared before. We close the cavity with the help of wooden sticks. Then, we place the chicken in a bowl with olive oil, and with a brush, we also smear the rest of the skin. We introduce the source in an oven at 190 degrees for approximately 1 hour and a half.

TENDERLOIN

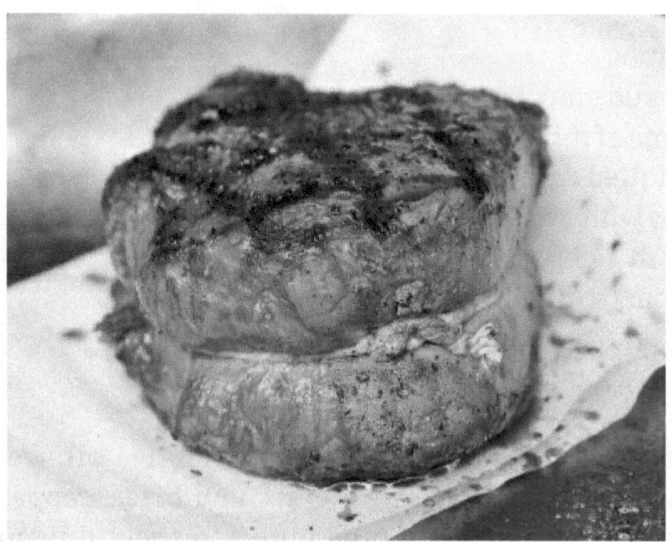

Ingredients:
400 grams of tenderloin in sabanitas of cream
Cheese
biscuit flour
virgin olive oil
Salt
We buy or ask the carnicera to make loin booklets that are nothing more than double fillets. We fill them with one or two sabanitas of cream cheese and close with chopsticks.

We heat abundant virgin olive oil in a pan and while batter the booklets in biscuit flour. When the oil is very hot, we introduce the booklets to brown. We must be careful that the inside of the booklets is well done since being double, we run the risk that the exterior is well made or at risk of burning, and the interior is raw.

FILLED CALAMARES

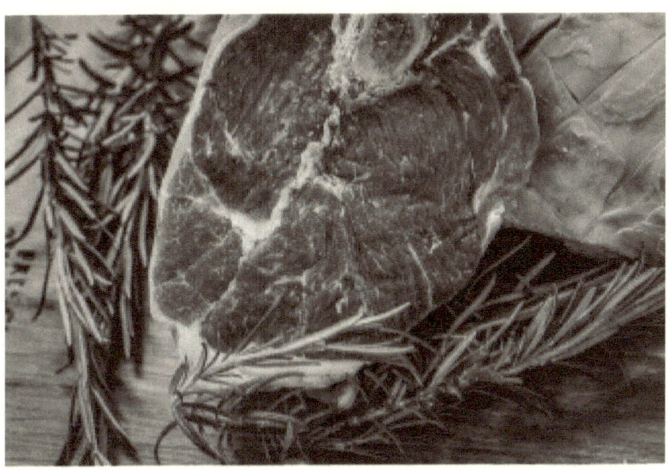

Ingredients:
1 medium or large squid per person
200 grams of minced meat green olives
boneless pine nuts
onion
ripe tomato green
pepper
1 glass of white wine
salt
black pepper
virgin olive oil
Peel and wash the squid reserving the tentacles.

In a pan with two tablespoons of virgin olive oil, we fry the minced meat by adding salt and ground black pepper. When it takes color, we incorporate the pine nuts, olives, and tentacles. We take the squids and start filling them with the minced meat mixture. When they are full, we close them with the help of a wooden stick.

In a clay pot, we make a stir-fry of green pepper, onion, and chopped tomatoes. We deposit the stuffed squid in the sofrito and sprinkle with white wines and a little salt. We put in the oven at 180 degrees, and in half an hour, they are ready to consume.

COD WITH AIOLI

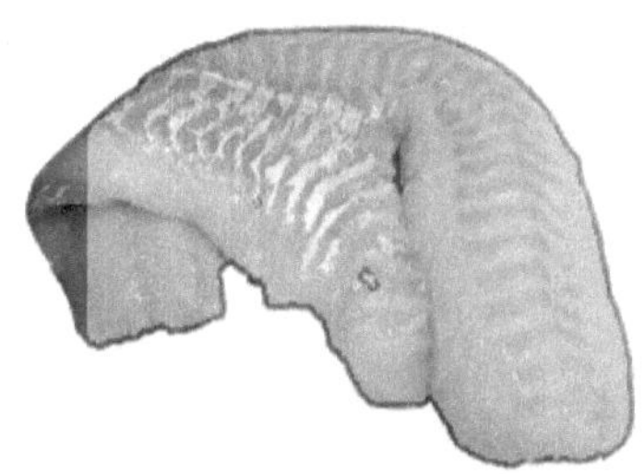

Ingredients:
Desalted cod loins with virgin olive oil skin – aioli (virgin olive oil and garlic)

Heat a pan for grilling with a few drops of oil. When it is very hot, we put the cod loins on the skin. We let the grill mark and separate it with a wooden spatula. While we will make the aioli with virgin olive oil and garlic, although it is no heresy to buy it made.

With the aioli, we cover the part of the loin that we have not gone through the iron. We put the loins in a bowl and take it to the oven, where we will keep it in gratin for about 10 minutes. The loins are usually served alone or accompanied by a sauce.

GRILLED LAMB

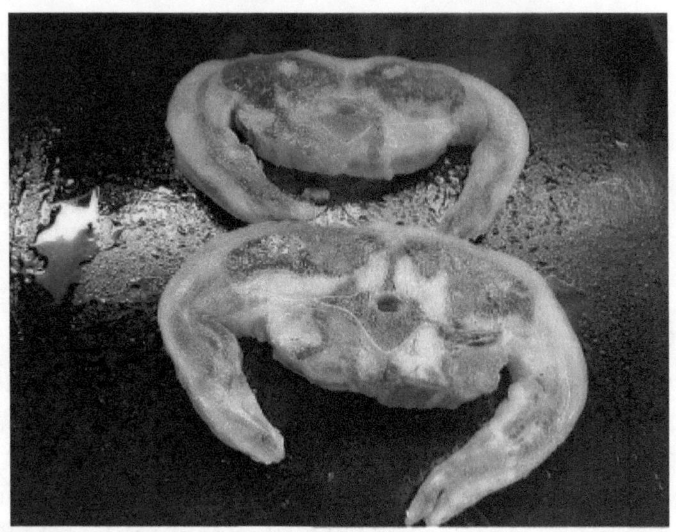

Ingredients:
6 or 8 fillets a lamb leg or chops of kidney stick
salt
virgin olive oil
chopped parsley chopped
garlic
black pepper powder
We heat a grill with a few drops of olive oil.
We deposit the pieces of meat salpimetlaslas and incorporating the chopped parsley and a little garlic powder. When the meat is still undercooked, we will turn around and repeat the seasoning. Grilled lamb meat should not be squeezed as it loses the juice and is very hard. Nor and for the same reason should it be overcooked. It should be slightly pink inside.

POULTRY FILLETS

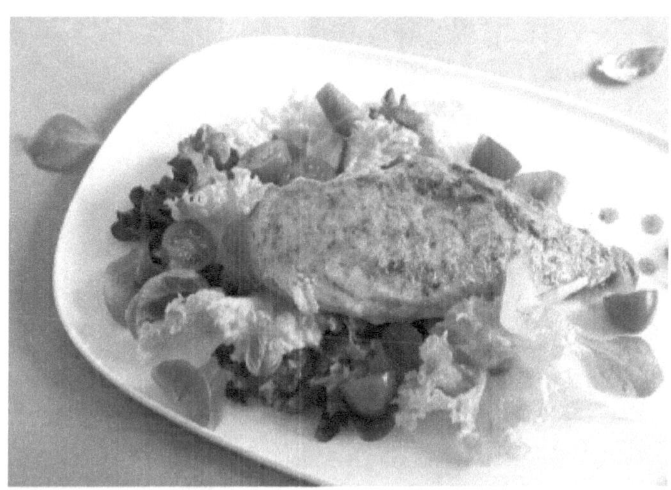

INGREDIENT:

Chicken or turkey breast fillets

biscuit flour or egg wheat (optional)

salt

parsley(optional)

garlic (optional)

We wash the steaks and dip them in a beaten egg. Then we batter them in a mixture of biscuit flour or wheat with salt. It is also possible to add chopped parsley and garlic to the mixture. In a pan with plenty of virgin olive oil, we fry the fillets until golden brown.

The use of eggs from our point of view blackens the oil very quickly and adds an extra protein that the meat does not need. And speaking of the flours, we prefer a biscuit flour rather than a wheat flour that we must "cook" along with the fillets. In any case, it is a matter of personal taste.

LAMB TO THE OVEN

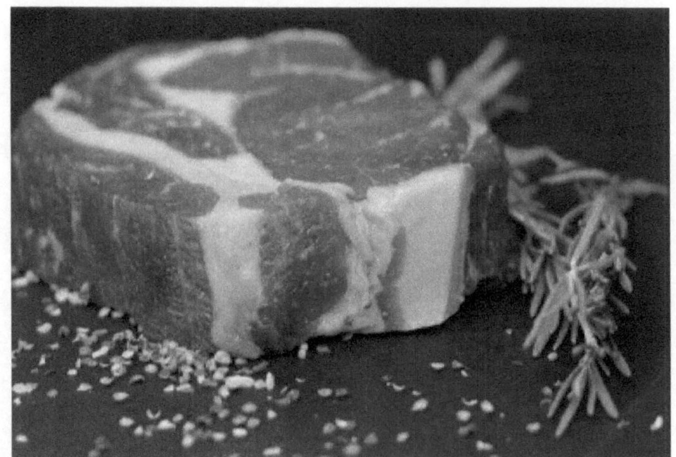

The lamb can be cooked "by itself" thanks to the amount of fat it contains. It can be baked from a leg of lamb to a modest serving of leg fillets. To know the time that must remain in the oven, we will look at the amount of grease of the piece. The fat will melt and help cooking in general. If, for example, we choose lamb leg fillet, it does not have too much fat, and we must add olive oil in greater proportion than if we used stick ribs.

INGREDIENTS
6 or 8 onion lamb leg fillets
garlic
virgin olive oil
salt and ground black pepper
1 glass of wine or water

In a flat clay pot, we put olive oil and brown a head of garlic and a large onion in rings over low heat. We put out the fire. Add the meat, salt, and pepper and optionally add a glass of wine or water. We adjust the oven to 180 degrees and leave the lamb until it is perceived done (this can vary and become up to 2 hours if the piece that was chosen were the whole leg instead of the fillets).

WRAPPED HONEY

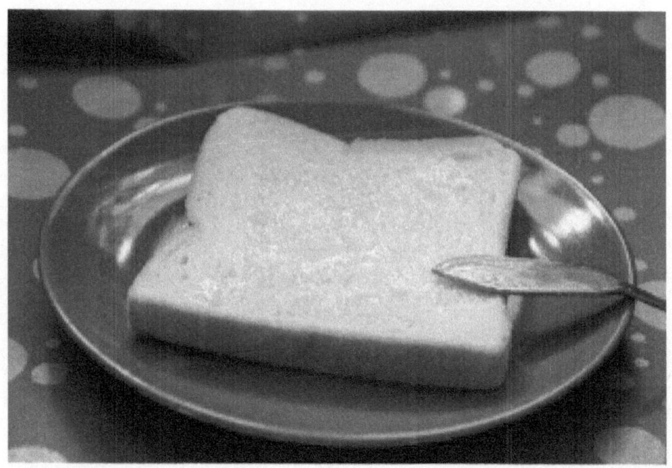

Melva is a fish of great nutritional value "belittled" by users and "mistreated" in fishmongers, where it usually does not exceed 3 euros per kilogram. It can be a substitute for tuna in samfainas or grilled. This is a really simple recipe to make.

Ingredients:

Melva (according to number of diners)

2 large purple onions

virgin olive oil

white wine

salt

In a pan with olive oil, sauté all the onion cut into rings, preventing it from burning. We can add a little salt to make the onion sweat. The onion should be beaten and a little golden. Place the sliced Melva on an onion bed and cover with the rest. We pour white wine until it covers the fish (1 glass should be enough). We put on low heat covering the pan, and in half an hour should be ready.

SEA TREAT

Ingredients:
Seabass according to the number of guests
Potatoes
Ripe tomatoes
Purple onion
Garlic
Parsley
Salt
Ground pepper
Virgin olive oil

In a container that can go to the oven and that we will have previously bathed in olive oil, we assemble a "bed" composed of onion rings and sliced potatoes that should cover the entire bottom. We also sliced unpeeled tomatoes. We pour a glass of water, wine or fish broth, salt, and pepper and put it in the oven at 180 degrees until the potatoes are soft. Then we place the fish on the bed of vegetables, sprinkling it with oil, salt, and chopped garlic with parsley. If the casserole is very dry, we will put another glass of liquid. We will keep for 20 minutes. The whole sea bass is served per diner (if they are very large, half) accompanied by the ration with potatoes and vegetables. If you want, you can add biscuit flour and gratin a few minutes before finishing the dish.

ZARZUELA FISH AND MARISCO EXPRESS

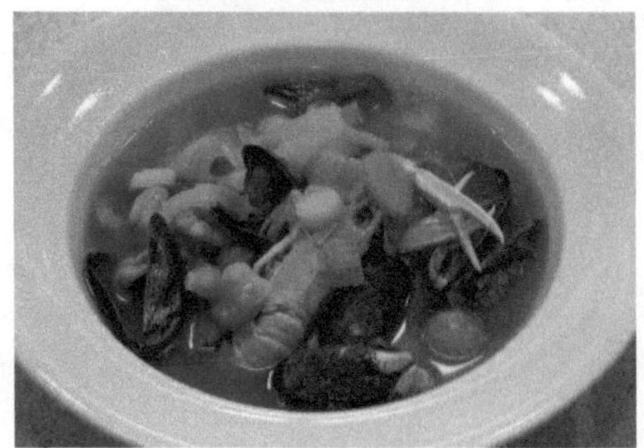

The title that I have given to this recipe is a bit misleading because the zarzuela of fish and seafood should always be express since the cooking times of both products are really very short. And if you do not do so, you will find that the fish crumbs and the seafood soften, ruining the presentation. The preparation time is about 20 minutes, half an hour at most. Another thing is the cost of the recipe that will depend on many factors: the type of fish you use, whether it is frozen or fresh.

Ingredients (4 people):
4 slices of monkfish (small / medium)
4 slices of hake (medium)
12 squid rings
8 prawns (if you put peeled prawns that are 12)
4 crayfish
16 mussels
2 large onions
3 ripe tomatoes
1 glass of white wine parsley fish stock
2 cloves garlic 4/5 almonds salt

black pepper virgin olive oil

We wash seafood and fish slices well. Now we are going to "pre-cook" some of them to speed up the preparation. In a pan with olive oil, lightly fry the slices of hake, squid rings, and monkfish previously floured. We preserve. In a flat clay pan (if possible) and using the fish frying oil, we will make a stir-fry with the two very finely chopped onions. We will pepper. When they begin to brown, we will add the tomatoes without skin or very chopped seeds, and when everything acquires texture, we will incorporate the glass of wine. We will let it be done until the liquid reduces.

While we will have made fish stock with remains of shrimp heads and some rockfish. If we do not have that possibility because the fish is frozen, we can use a ready-made fish broth or even a pill. We must make a total of half a liter of broth. When the sauce is reduced, we will add the hot broth and then all the fish simmering for a maximum of 10 minutes. Five minutes before the end, we will add the seafood. We will take the opportunity to make a chopped with parsley, two garlic heads, and four almonds, incorporating it in half cooking. We will rectify salt. With those ten minutes is more than enough. The zarzuela broth will remain liquid, and it will only be enough to serve a couple of tablespoons as a bottom of the dish, distributing the fish evenly. If we want the broth to be thicker, we can add wheat flour - 1 tablespoon

-previously cooked (just fry it in a little oil) or simply add fried bread to the chop.

BAKED SALMONETES

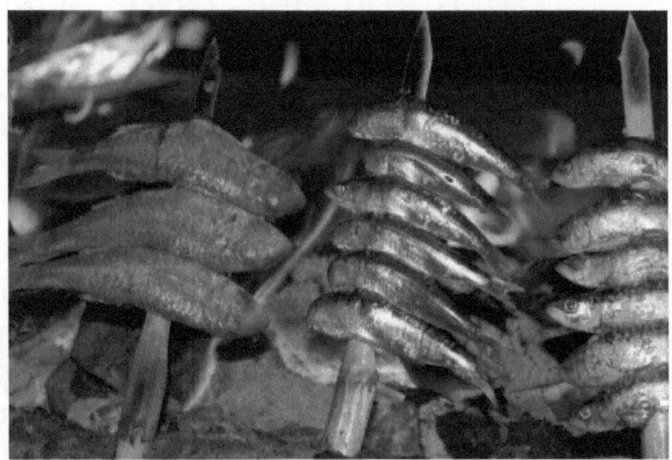

I present a fish of "second category" that, in my opinion, is one of the tastiest that can be found. There are two types, the mud, and the rock, although personally, I prefer the second. To distinguish one from the other, you must note that the rock has a dark line that goes from the eye to the tail and is crossed by yellow stripes while the mud is a uniform color. This recipe is very quick to make and really cheap.

Ingredients:

Rock mullets (depending on the number of diners) or mud, as you find ripe tomato

parsley

cookie flour or breadcrumbs salt

garlic

black pepper

a glass of white wine

virgin olive oil

In a refractory tray to go to the oven, we place the fish without guts and clean. Salpimentamos. Peel and remove the seeds from the tomatoes to chop them very finely. We do the same with garlic cloves, parsley, and cookie flour. Then we pour virgin olive oil and the wine on top. We put in the oven at 180 degrees for half an hour (or until we see that they are made). They are served as is or accompanied by half a lemon to finish dressing. The mullet is the type of fish that even people who do not like fish generally like, so it is a good "initiatory" dish.

COCA

Coca is very typical of the gastronomy of Lleida, although, at present, it can be found throughout Catalonia, mainly for sale in traditional bread ovens. Its form and ingredients are reminiscent of pizza, and in fact, it seems that it appears in the fifteenth or sixteenth century thanks to the cultural interaction between the Kingdom of Aragon and its possessions in southern Italy. On which one preceded which other is difficult to determine, although the immense popularity of pizza will certainly prevent the "minority" recapte coca from being considered the mother of this culinary specialty.

The preparation is very simple, especially if you choose to buy a dough already prepared to put in the oven. To prepare the garnish, we will do exactly the same as to prepare scalding if we opt for a totally vegetable option. It is also very common to make meat cocas by adding sausage or botifarra and even fish with the addition of a harangue. I will also give you the recipe for the dough, which is not difficult to make but takes time.

Ingredients for Coca:
1/2 kg wheat flour
3 tablespoons butter
30 grams of yeast
1/2 virgin olive oil 1 glass of warm water
Salt

Ingredients for Guarnition:
1 large onion
2 or 3 red peppers
1 eggplant
2 ripe tomatoes

2 or 3 botifarras

First, we will do the scalding. We use a microwave resistant glass or ceramic container where we will deposit the vegetables if possible, whole. If this is not possible, we will cut them into longitudinal strips of the largest possible size; otherwise, it would be very difficult to peel them. Once we have arranged the vegetables in the bowl, we will bathe them in abundant virgin olive oil. We will use the microwave at a power of 700 W for 45 minutes. You may notice that the vegetables swell during cooking. This in itself is not worrisome, but we must make sure that they do not burn, which can occur if any vegetable is exposed to the microwave without being covered with oil. In the event that the volume of the vegetable pile is not possible for all of them to be bathed, we will give them a review of oil with a brush. When the relevant 45 minutes have elapsed, we will remove the container, and under the tap stream, we will cool the vegetables one by one. a. The skin will have cracked and separated from the meat, being easy to peel the tomatoes, peppers in addition to the eggplant. We will open the peppers and tomatoes to remove all the seeds while in the eggplant, we will extract the most that we can, since trying it all would be impossible. Cut the vegetables into thin strips, add more virgin olive oil and salt according to taste.

Now we will prepare the dough if that is our option. First, we put the flour on the marble of the kitchen, making a "mountain" and make a hole in the center. In that hole, we put the water, the yeast, the salt, and the butter and work it until it doesn't stick to the stone. When this happens, we cover it with a cloth and leave for at least three hours to ferment. After three hours, we return to work the dough this time, adding the oil little by little until it is completely dissolved in the dough.

Finally, we will compose the coca. For this, we will flour a container that can go to the oven where we will put the dough, giving it the desired shape. On top of it, we will put the scalded drained cut into strips (eggplant and peppers) and rings the onion. We will also place botifarras. With the same oil of the scalded, we slightly wet the surface and put a little salt on the meat. We put the oven at 180 degrees and keep the coca inside for about 30 minutes or until we see it done. It can be consumed hot or cold. Obviously, like pizza, coca allows the fantasy we want in terms of the garnish, although the one described, the vegetable and the one containing sandwiches are the traditional ones.

RAJADA DELETE

Ibiza, apart from beaches and discos, has rich gastronomy that is worth checking out. It has both sea and mountain dishes and that should not surprise us because the islands are microcosms that are reordered as miniature continents: for the locals the distances that seem continental to us are ridiculous they seem insurmountable and speak of the people of the interior - an interior that is not usually beyond 10 kilometers of the coast - as of different cultural entities. Ibiza is a good example of this. We have powerful dishes made exclusively with farmyard products and excellent fish dishes, among which the Borrida de Rajada stand out. La Rajada is La Raya in Spanish, in general, a very cheap fish that has been traditionally belittled by both consumers and fishermen. In my way of understanding, the line is a fish with a very fine flavor with the added attraction of some edible cartilage that crosses it from side to side. Regarding the recipe I am going to give, it is important to clarify that there is a "prior" that consists of marinating the line in salt and lemon juice. This prior was aimed at eliminating a hypothetical aroma of ammonia that gave off meat, something that in my opinion, only occurs with certain fish, especially sharks, when the meat is not in very good condition. To this day, I have never noticed that aroma in any conveniently fresh stripe, but I keep the marinade of the recipe because I believe that some connoisseur will not seem the same flavor without the powerful lemon aroma.

Ingredients:

4 or 5 pieces of stripe

About 1 Kg lemons

salt

2 garlic cloves

fried almonds
2 slices of toasted bread or fried parsley sprig
1 egg
virgin olive oil
Marinate the line for about 3 or 4 hours in water with plenty of salt and lemon juice. At the end of the process, we take out the pieces, pass them through the water. Then we put them in just water and boil until the stripe is half cooked. Again, we discard the cooking water and put new water where we will continue cooking the stripe over moderate or slow heat.

Now we will prepare the dressing. We will put the garlic and fried almonds in a mortar, add salt and crush. Then we add the parsley and toasted bread. Finally, we shell an egg and mix it with the dough with a drizzle of olive oil. This mixture is incorporated into the line by sprinkling it over, and it only remains to be done over low heat. From my point of view and to accelerate the preparation, you can skip the theme of the marinade, especially if you have not prepared this dish before and, therefore, do not have a "memory" of the flavor.

So you can see that Ibiza is more than just a party beach.

DUCK

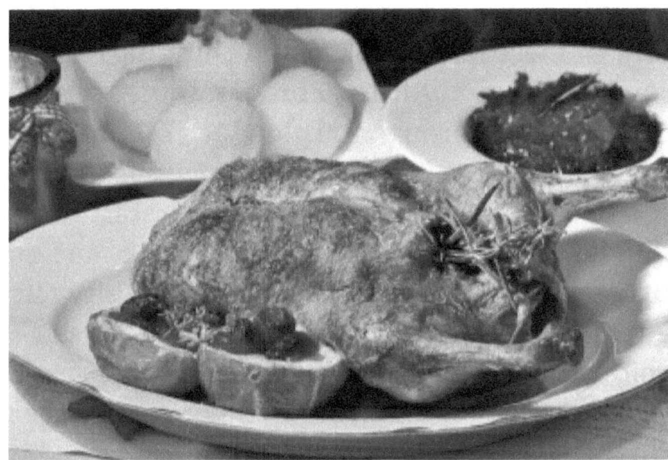

The duck is a bird whose meat is much leatherier than chicken and therefore requires high cooking times. This recipe combines what would be a roast duck with a special broth where we will just soften the meat. I just cooked and ate one of these - specifically a thigh - so I have all the details extremely fresh in my mind.

Ingredients:

1 magret or duck leg (per diner)

1 leek

2 large carrots

1 purple onion ("Figueres" type)

1 garlic clove

1/4 of a glass of red wine

salt

virgin olive oil

First, we will brown the thigh or magret in a pan with olive oil. It is simply to mark the piece and give some flavor to the oil, not to cook it. We preserve in the oil that we have used for the meat we lightly fry a clove of garlic, and when it is lightly golden, we will add the leek, carrot, and onion cut in julienne already with the live fire. We will add salt so that the vegetables give off water. When this kind of sofrito has acquired texture, and the onion has expired, we will incorporate vegetable broth, preferably, and, if not, simply water. The quantity of broth or water should range between half and one liter since it will depend on the amount of meat to be cooked and thinking that the liquid should cover the pieces. After 15 or 20 minutes of cooking, we pass all the elements through the blender (it is not necessary to make a fine puree). Now is the time to introduce the meat that should be bathed. We will lower the heat and start slow cooking that should last for at least an hour. A quarter of an hour before the end of the planned cooking time, we will rectify salt and add the stream of red wine. Let's be cautious with the salt since the purple onion and the leek tend to make a sweet sauce, and no matter how much salt we put, we will not rectify that characteristic. In the end, we will have the soft meat bathed in a sauce with excellent flavor and texture.

If at the end of the process the meat is not as soft as we want it to be - always keep in mind that the duck is not chicken - we can add a teaspoon of vinegar to soften.

SNAILS WITH HAM

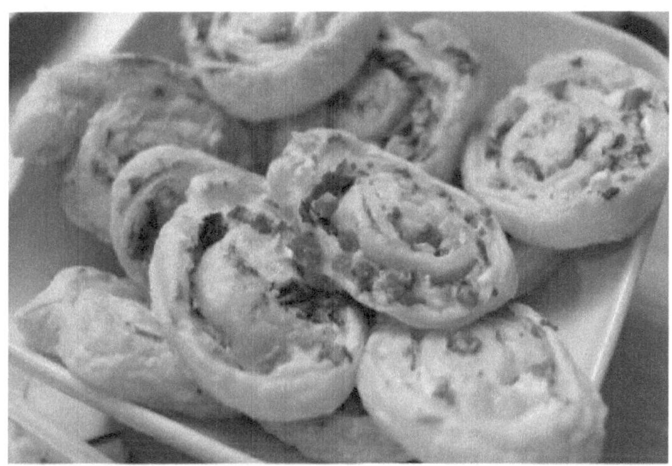

An extremely simple recipe to prepare succulent snails.
Ingredients:
1 Kg of clean snails
onion
ripe tomato
garlic
black pepper
virgin olive oil
wheat flour
salt
Iberian ham in tacos
If we have live snails that have not yet been washed, we will first proceed to purify them for at least 48 hours. For this, we will put them in a bucket with abundant saltwater with vinegar. We will change the water several times. Finally, we will put them in a pot that we will put on low heat. When the water is hot, the snails will have removed a blackish substance. Then, remove from heat and wash with plenty of cold water. It is also possible

to buy already clean, precooked, and even frozen snails.

In a flat clay pot, we will make a stir-fry with 1 onion, 2 ripe tomatoes and a clove of garlic. We will pour a couple of tablespoons of wheat flour and work it to cook it. We toss the small sliced Iberian ham tacos. We fry them with the rest of the ingredients. Then we will pour 1/2 liter of water, salt, and black pepper in abundance (must be quite spicy). Finally, we will incorporate the snails constantly removing them so that they are soaked in the broth, and obviously, they are soft.

RUSSIAN BISTEC

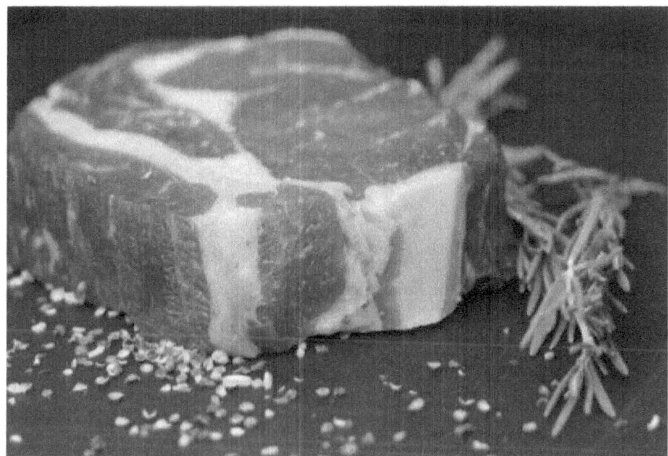

I do not know what the origin of the Russian steak is, but I suspect that it comes from Russia and could be related to the steak tartar that the Tartars consumed, a very spicy minced meat that was obviously eaten raw. Somehow, he arrived in Germany, and there he began to fry and then go to the United States where he would become, very modified, the hamburger we all know (hamburger for being carried by German emigrants from that city). In summary, the steak tartar would have given rise to the American hamburger, the Russian steak, and various variants that are still consumed in Germany.

Ingredients:

400 grams of beef or minced pork

1 egg

2 garlic heads

parsley breadcrumbs

salt

ground black pepper

wheat flour

virgin olive oil
milk (optional)
In a bowl, mix the minced meat with garlic and very finely chopped parsley. Beat the egg and add it with a handful of breadcrumbs, salt, and pepper. We work the mixture until it is as homogeneous as possible. If we perceive what remains to be very dry, add a little milk. With the hand, we grab a dough ball, smash it into the kitchen marble, and flatten it. Generally, the height is 1 cm, and it is made somewhat larger than a "traditional" hamburger.
Flour the resulting steaks and fry in abundant virgin olive oil. If they have been a little raw inside but externally, they start to blacken it is better to take them out of the pan and finish the preparation in the oven, about 180º for approximately 15 minutes.
It is served with vegetables, steamed rice, etc.

RABBIT WITH VINAGRETA DE PIÑONES

The rabbit is one of the healthiest meats we can taste. It is often eaten grilled, and although it is really very good, it has always seemed to me that it was a bit dry. With the addition of a hot pineapple vinaigrette, this sensation disappears.

Ingredients:

1 chopped rabbit

50 grams of pine nuts

laurel

olive oil (1/2 cup)

wine vinegar

salt

black pepper

In a metallic casserole, we will arrange the rabbit pieces so that they all fit without piling up but without too much slack. That is, we will try to make the casserole size fit the meat. We will add pepper. We will incorporate half a glass of virgin olive oil or a little more if we see that it is not enough to make the vinaigrette sauce a posteriori and a bay leaf. We will throw the pine nuts and put them on very low heat with the saucepan covered. We will leave about an hour for the rabbit to be done and remove from heat. We extract the pieces of meat and place them in a very hot pan to make grilled. While they are done, we will add one or two tablespoons of wine vinegar (depending on how much we like vinegar sauces) and remove the bay leaf. Add a little salt. Heat the pan again for a couple of minutes, stirring the mixture, and the vinaigrette is ready.

We serve the grilled rabbit watering it with the vinaigrette on the side or on the side so that the diner soaks the meat to your liking.

HAM CROQUETTES

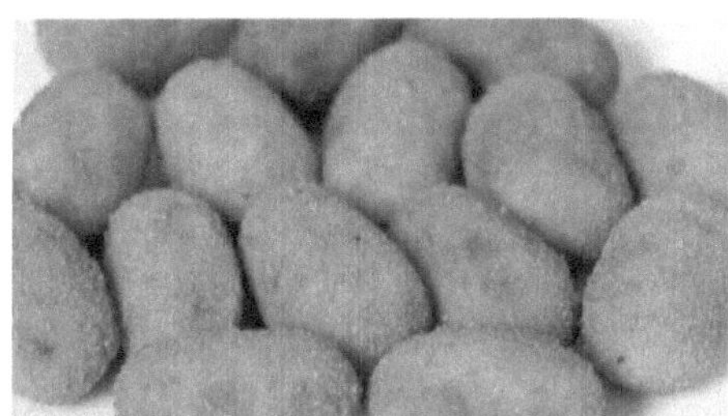

A croquette is basically a fairly solidified bechamel that has been shaped to fry it later. The taste of bechamel is quite simple, so it is customary to incorporate more palatable products such as chicken, tuna, and, as in the recipe at hand, ham.

Ingredients:

purple onion type "Figueres"

garlic

wheat flour

butter

1 liter of whole milk

cured ham

salt

virgin olive oil

In a saucepan, we pour the oil and fry the chopped onion with a clove of garlic. When the onion is expired, add the ham in small pieces and put a very low heat. Remove the garlic and add a good spoon of butter and melting another wheat flour. We work with a spoon or some rods so that the sauce is binding. We begin to incorporate the milk little by little. When the dough is already bound and does not stop for more, we continue adding more butter, flour, and milk without stopping working with the spoon. We must calculate the number of ingredients according to the number of croquettes we want. We will take salt and go checking that the flavor moves away from the taste of raw flour and takes the flavor of ham. Let it cold down. We separate dough balls and work it to obtain the cylindrical shape of the croquettes. Flour and fry in plenty of oil. You have to be careful with the salt since the ham incorporates enough, and with the heat, it accentuates it even more.

FIDEUÀ

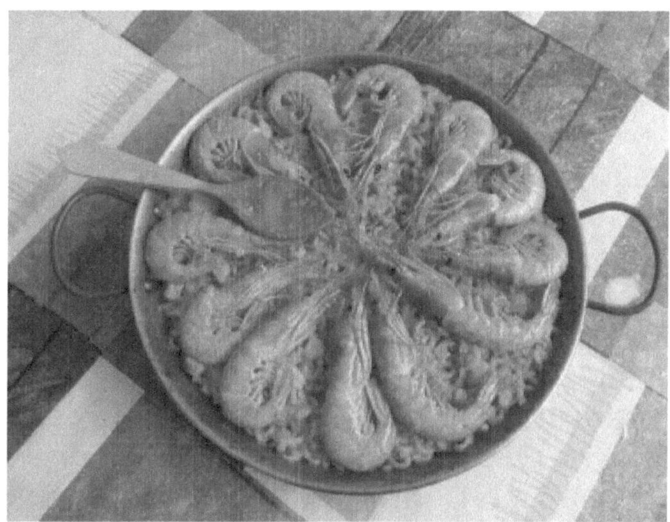

Fideuà is similar to seafood or fish rice replacing rice with noodles. The legend says that he was born when some fishermen from Gandia wanted to make rice on the high seas and realized that they had forgotten it. They then took hold of what they had available, specifically a package of noodles.

Ingredients:

A package of 250-gram noodles

3 gauge

1 purple onion, type "figueres"

1 clove garlic

2 or 3 ripe tomatoes sweet paprika (optional)

Various seafood (prawns, crayfish, mussels, etc.)

Fish (monkfish, grouper, etc.)

Water

fish stock

saffron

We make a stir-fry with the onion and garlic chopped very, very finely. We will eat when the onion expires, and before it burns, we will throw the peeled tomato cut, also very thin. Let it simmer until it takes texture.

As it is done with rice, we then sauté the noodles, although, for a much shorter time than what we used for rice. We heat the fish stock, and when it boils, we pour it on the stir-fry and the noodles. Remember that the water or broth to be incorporated must be twice as much as the paste used. If we have a glass of noodles, we will use two glasses of broth. This is important because the fideuà must be wet but without broth (or really very little).

The time to pour the broth is also to incorporate the spices if we have them, specifically paprika and saffron. If not, we will look at the infinity with a landscape face.

We throw salt again. Unlike rice, pasta is not very critical about salt. We rise to live fire. When we foresee that the pasta is going to be made, we throw the seafood and the fish that together should not cook more than five minutes. I hope you have at least some seafood no matter how humble it is, and you can park the landscape face. The fideuà is ready to be consumed.

MUSAKA

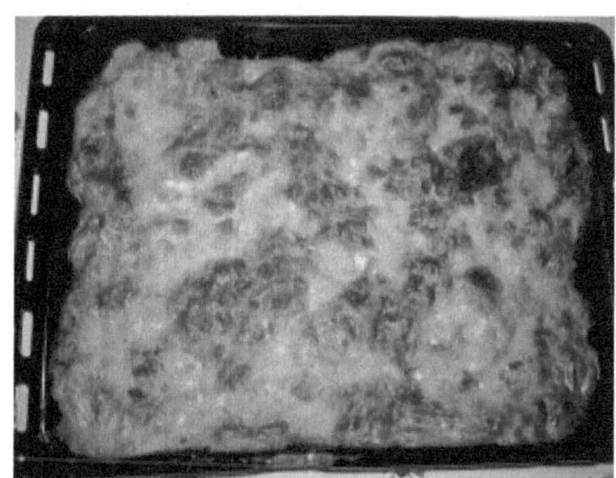

Greek musaka is similar to lasagna, although using eggplant instead of pasta. It is a very strong dish as the Greeks prepare it since it uses lamb meat that is very fatty.

Ingredients:

1 Kg of minced lamb meat (you can use veal or pork)

2 large eggplants

1 large onion

8 ripe tomatoes (approximately 1 kg of tomatoes)

Wheat flour

Milk

salt

oregano

black pepper

nutmeg

grated cheese

olive oil

Prepare the eggplants by cutting them into thin slices. We add enough salt and place them in a bowl of water for half an hour to lose the bitter taste.

We prepare the tomato sauce. First, we will peel and remove the seeds from the tomatoes. Then we fry the chopped onion, and when it begins to brown, we will add the tomatoes with a spoonful of salt. We will cover and let it acquire texture. We preserve.

We take the eggplants and dry them with a paper towel or cloth. They must be very dry. Then we fry them in olive oil until they brown. We let them rest in a paper that sucks the excess oil.

We take the minced meat and fry it by adding salt and black pepper. It should not be completely done since we will finish the recipe in the oven.

Finally, we will prepare the bechamel. To do this, we will have two tablespoons of olive oil in a metallic saucepan and add the wheat flour. We will stir with a whisk to break the flour. While stirring, add the milk and a pinch of salt until it begins to thicken. If we wish we will grate a little nutmeg. We preserve.

Now, it remains to mount the moussaka in the refractory vessel that will go to the oven. First of all, we will spread some tomato sauce at the bottom. Then, the minced meat and on it in order another bit of fried tomato, oregano, and eggplants. If we have a lot of each ingredient, we can make a second floor in the same order. Otherwise, we will close by pouring fried tomato on the eggplants and the béchamel sauce. We will sprinkle grated cheese on the set.

We will put the oven at 180º, letting the moussaka be done for about 20 minutes. After that time, we will grate until the cheese is golden brown.

CHAPTER 7 - DESSERTS

RICE WITH MILK

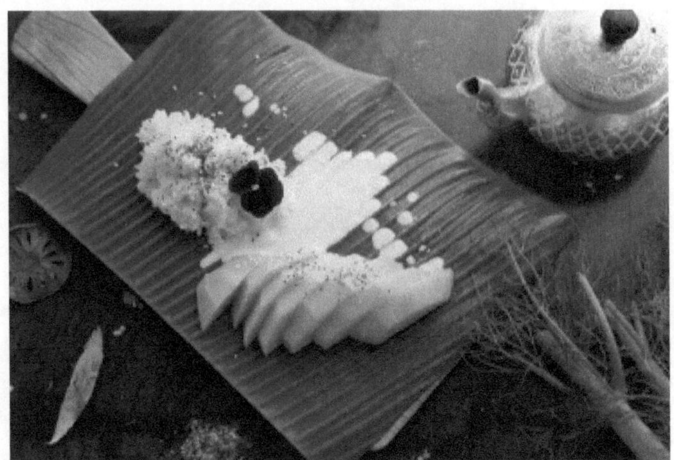

Ingredients:

½ liter of whole or semi-skimmed milk

50 grams of rice

50 grams of sugar

1 lemon peel

1 cinnamon stick cinnamon powder

Peel the lemon to obtain a strip of skin, taking care not to take the white part of it since it is bitter. Therefore, the peeling should be slightly transparent.

Add the skin and cinnamon sticks to ½ liter of milk and heat it while stirring until it boils. We will watch so that at that time, the saucepan does not overflow and immediately reduce the fire. We will add the rice and sugar constantly stirring so that it does not stick to the bottom. Occasionally, we will try some grain of rice to check that it is soft. When the rice is done, we will remove from the heat and let stand until it is warm. Then we will pour the contents into small containers for direct consumption or in a large container that will go directly to the refrigerator. When it has cooled, it will be ready for consumption by adding a little cinnamon powder to the diner's taste.

MACEDONIA OF FRUITS

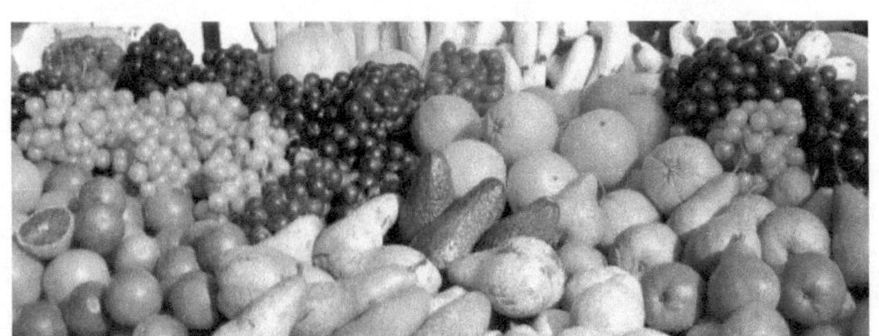

Ingredients:

2 kiwifruits

2 table oranges

6/8 juice oranges

2 apples

2 vine peaches

2 bananas

1 pineapple

1 unsweetened plain yogurt (optional)

We squeeze the oranges to get the juice.

We filter and deposit it in a bowl.

Peel and cut the kiwis, apples, pineapple, and peaches into small tacos. We incorporate the juice. We cut the two table oranges into slices and then into easy-to-take segments. We will make slices of bananas. We will not mix or add sugar of any kind (the fruit has fructose that is the natural and own sweetener). If you are not going to consume the fruit salad immediately, it is advisable to mix two tablespoons of plain yogurt with some rods to slow down the oxidation.

STRAWBERRIES IN ENGLISH CREAM

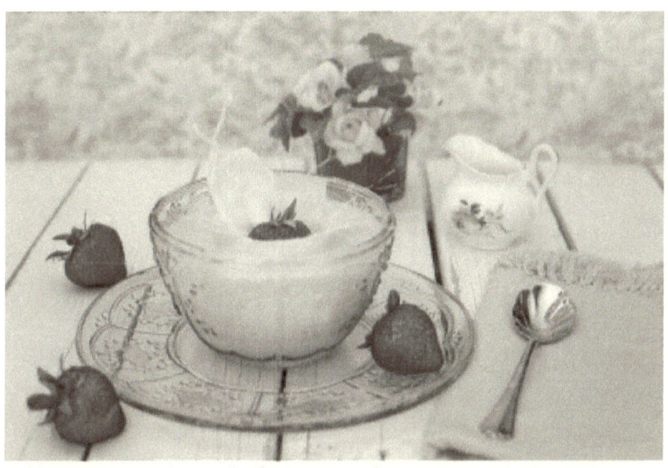

It is a really exceptional dessert that you can serve on special occasions.

Ingredients:

Fresones according to the number of guests (1/2 Kg approx.)

1/2-liter semi-skimmed milk 125 grams sugar

4 eggs

1 branch of vanilla

Bring the milk to a boil to reduce the heat to a minimum below. We take only the yolks of the four eggs and beat them with the sugar with the rod mixer. We add the yolks and the vanilla branch to the milk. We raise the heat a little and do not stop stirring for ten minutes. We will watch so that the milk does not boil at any time.

Remove from heat, and when the temperature drops and then, after some time, we cool it in the fridge.

We wash the strawberries and, without being too big, we split them. We place in an ice-cream cup and bathe just before serving with the English cream. As it is served with a lot of creams and it is very liquid, a spoon should be used, and therefore the strawberry pieces should be adapted to this fact (we cannot let the diners be forced to chop the fruit with the edge of the spoon).

PAN GREIXONERA

This recipe is a variation of the well-known Ibizan dessert called Greixonera. In this dessert, hard ensaimadas from previous days are used. Due to the difficulty of finding such raw material, it is possible to use hard bread instead of ensaimadas. The results are quite good, and we also give out that hard bread that stays in our houses, this time in the form of dessert. The ingredients that I indicate are for two portions.

Ingredients:
4 slices of bread
1/4-liter milk (just over a glass)
1 egg
75 grams of sugar
cinnamon powder
lemon
virgin olive oil

We boil the milk with a little lemon peel. When it has taken the first boil, we will remove from the heat, removing the skin of the lemon. While we will lightly fry the slices of bread in olive oil, remove them before they are burned, to place them on absorbent paper, and thus remove the excess oil. With the milk still very hot, we will incorporate the sugar and dissolve it. Then, immediately deposit the slices of bread at the bottom of the container, if possible, without stacking them.

Sprinkle ground cinnamon on the slices. Let stand about 10 minutes so that the bread is soaked in milk. If, after ten minutes, there is no milk left, we will add a little since the consistency of the dough should be pasty but not dry. Now we will proceed to shred the bread with the help of a fork or a rod mixer. It should not be excessively fine, so do not use the electric mixer. Once this is done, we beat an egg and incorporate it, mixing it well with the rest of the ingredients. It only remains to put in the oven previously heated to 180 degrees for exactly half an hour. The dough rises but very slightly; do not expect it to sponge as if it had yeast. In any case, when cooling, it will return to take the volume it had before baking. It is put in the fridge when it has reached room temperature, and in about six hours, when it is very cold, it is ready to consume. In spite of what it may seem, it does not taste "to bread" but rather to a sweet made with flan.

The total time of realization is about 45 minutes, and it is a dessert "that always comes out," even if the number of diners varies. If there were, for example, 8 people, we would need to simply multiply by 4 the milk, bread, and sugar used here, and the result would be the same.

FLOATING ISLAND

To better understand this dessert, it is possible to say that it is a flan made with egg white that "floats" on a somewhat diluted Catalan cream. Or a meringue over custard, as preferred. All this said with tweezers so that purists do not put their hands to their heads.

Ingredients:

1/2 liter of milk

6 eggs

500 grams of sugar Essence of vanilla or branch 1 pinch of salt

First, we will make the cream. We will heat the milk. Beat the egg yolks with 100 grams of sugar, then add the hot milk and vanilla. We stir for about 10 minutes without ever letting it boil. Remove and let cool.

Now we will beat the egg whites that we have separated with the 200 grams of sugar and the pinch of salt to the point of snow. We will prepare a candy with 200 grams of sugar and a glass of water. With the caramel still hot, we will bathe the inside of a flanera. Now we will put the clear whips in the flank, trying not to have any air left. Then we will put the flanera to the water bath in the oven for about 45 minutes (or until it feels tacky) to 180 degrees. We take out and unmold. We cool in the fridge.

When the cream and meringue are cold, we will proceed to assemble the dish. It's called a floating island because we make the meringue, which is very light, float on the cream. Therefore, at least we will use a bowl of soup that we will fill in its 3/4 parts with cream. Then we will cut a piece of meringue and put it in the center. It can be decorated with chocolate chips if desired.

PINEAPPLE BRUSH AND CATALAN CREAM

Ingredients:
1 liter of milk
4 egg yolks
200 grams of sugar
cinnamon
lemon bark
stick natural pineapple (or syrup)
First, we will make the Catalan cream. We will heat the milk with the cinnamon stick and the lemon rind. We will beat the yolks with the sugar, incorporating the hot milk, removing the cinnamon, and the lemon rind. We want to have a somewhat thick Catalan cream. To do this, we introduce it in the oven at 180 º to the water bath for about 12 minutes. If we spend time, we will have flan, and if we fall short, we will have cream too liquid, so we will monitor to remove when we have a midpoint.
We take out a slice of pineapple and cut it into tacos after having separated it from the peel. We will get between 6 and 8 sections. We take the metal or wooden skewer and skewer one after another, the sections that we have obtained from the pineapple slit. We take the cream still hot and pour it over the pineapple pieces, without exaggeration. We put a layer of sugar on the whole skewer and burn it with the help of a hot plate and if we do not have a metal spoon previously heated to the fire. We serve on the plate with an extra shovel of Catalan cream next to the skewer.

PEARS AND WINE

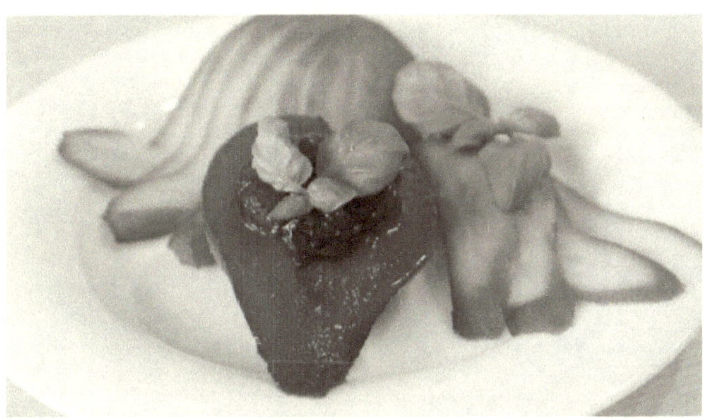

Ingredients:

4 (1 per diner) "hard" pears (approximately 1 Kg)

1/2 glass of red wine

1/2 glass of sugar

1 lemon rind

1 cinnamon stick

Peel the pears and place them in a small saucepan. Pears should be "tight" but not crammed on top of each other. We pour the wine incorporating the lemon rind (without the white part because bitter) and the cinnamon stick. We put on medium heat so that it is done slowly. The cooking time depends on the hardness of the pear but ranges between 10 and 20 minutes. After this time, we incorporate the sugar, and without stopping stirring, we keep about 15 minutes. If it becomes dry, we add a little more wine. They are served at room temperature bathed in a little broth.

It should be noted that whenever we use wine, it must be of quality. If we are not able to drink the wine we pour at meals, it is certain that these will not be good. Pears with wine is a traditional dessert of the Cantabrian coast.

SWEET MILK

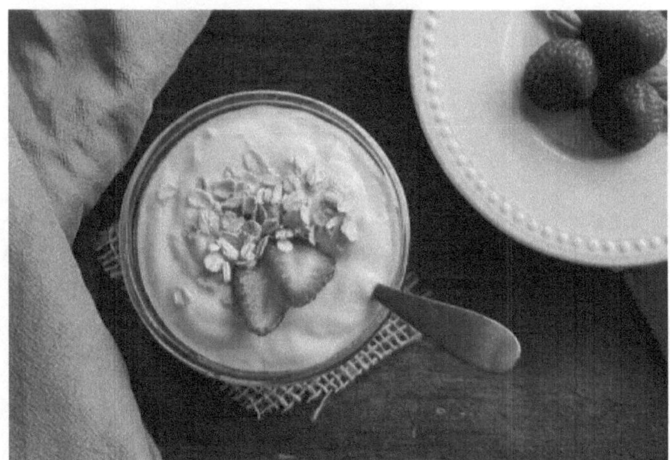

Dulce de leche is original from Argentina but very popular in practically all of South America. Its preparation is very simple, although due to the high sugar content, it is not advisable to abuse its consumption.

Ingredients:

1/2 liter of milk

125 grams of sugar

1 teaspoon of baking soda dissolved in half a glass of water

Add the milk and sugar in a saucepan over low heat stirring so that it mixes well. While stirring, add the water with the baking soda. To those who have missed this ingredient simply say that it serves to accelerate the caramelization process. We continue stirring until after passing the wooden spoon; you can see the bottom of the saucepan. Optionally you can incorporate vanilla essence.

Let it cool. The dulce de leche can be served as is or as a crepe filling, spread on bread or toast, etc.

TRADITIONAL GREIXONERA

Recipes that use hard bread or recycle by-products from other foods seem great to me as a sign of trust and above all because sometimes these derived foods are more surprising than the original ones. It is not often that we are faced with a recipe for a dessert that uses derivative products, in this case, hard ensaimadas, but there is. The greixonera is a very typical dessert of Ibiza that is practically found in the menus of all the restaurants on the island. It is very simple to make, and the taste is really exceptional.

Ingredients (for 2 people):
2 hard ensaimadas per medium-sized person
4 eggs (1 per ensaimada)
150 grams of sugar
1/2 liter of milk
lemon
butter
cinnamon powder

Cook the milk and let it cool. Then we beat the 4 eggs and add them. We make pieces with the ensaimadas and also incorporate them with the sugar and the grated lemon peel. Although it is not in the original recipe, I like to add a cinnamon stick and beat with a rod mixer to undo the piece of ensaimada, although without exaggeration. The mixture is put in the "greixonera" - which is not more than a flat clay casserole - which we have previously smeared with butter. Place in the oven for 1/2 hour at 180 degrees and serve it sprinkle with cinnamon powder. It is a real delicacy.

CHAPTER 8 - DRINKS

BLEEDING

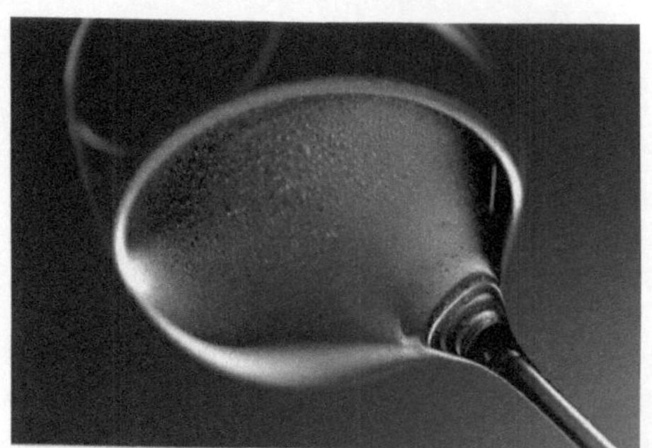

There are hundreds of sangria recipes. Some include mixtures of soft drinks with gas, high-grade spirits, and even cinnamon. This could be one of many.

Ingredients:
1 liter of quality red wine
2 juice oranges
2 peaches

sugar or liquid sweetener
The wine and juice of the two oranges are mixed in a jar. The peaches are cut into dice and incorporated. We try the mixture and add sugar until we get the flavor that we like. If we have difficulty dissolving sugar, we can use a liquid sweetener. We keep in the fridge and keep the maceration for at least 6 hours.

CHUFA HORCHATA

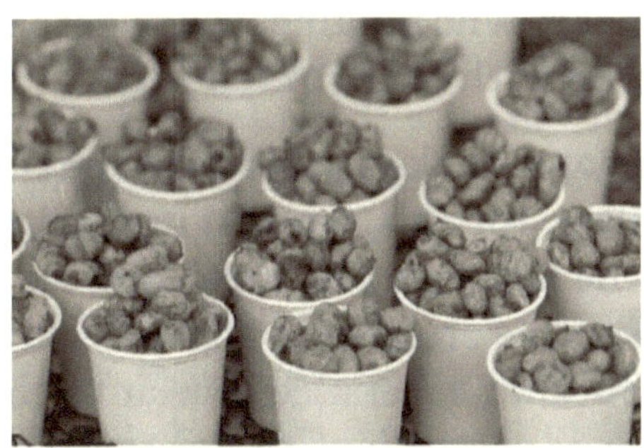

The consumption of certain products is strongly conditioned by the season of the year in which we are. This is the case with the gazpacho and horchata that live their moment of glory in summer to disappear from our diets the rest of the year. This is a shame because both products provide a substantial amount of nutrients and are so healthy that they deserve to be in our refrigerators from January to December.

Chufa horchata is produced from underground tubers that are obtained from a plant called hazelnut sedge. The process involves thorough washing of the chufa, crushing, and finally, the addition of water and sugar. We can buy the packaged chufa horchata, or we can make it ourselves. There is a big difference between the two. Apart from how natural it is, if we do it, the taste changes radically. To make chufa horchata, we will need:

500 grams of chufas
2 liters of bottled water
250 grams of sugar

The chufas are obtained in places of sale of nuts.

First of all, we must keep the chufas 24 hours to soak so that into nutritional faults; As an example, I will say that diabetics have to take care of these aspects very carefully since otherwise, they fall too often into malnutrition.

Finally, if you found this book useful in any way, a review on Amazon is always appreciated!